FOREWORD

FITNESS FIRST, in my view, answers the need for a book on human body structure, functions and mechanics, and explains in simple terms the jargon often associated with medical matters. No prior knowledge of the subject seems necessary and I am confident it will appeal to many groups of readers in whatever walk of life, from sports men and women, teachers and students, to nurses and even medical students, administrators and executives.

It is well illustrated by the author himself and with illustrations by eminent lecturers in physiology at the University of Glasgow which appear in McNaught and Callander's Illustrated Physiology. Each chapter is complete in itself, repeating information where necessary which avoids confusing and time consuming back references.

The text is well presented, based on factual evidence and is a useful handbook on how to achieve and maintain physical fitness and will prove invaluable as a learning and teaching aid.

Ruth M. Kirkham
KFA National Tutor Trainer
Chairman, The Keep Fit Association:
South West Region

ACKNOWLEDGMENTS

Present day knowledge of the human mind, body and nutrition owes much to the pioneers of Anatomy and Physiology and their established scientific facts. Facts are the ultimate truth which cannot change, are never contradictory and are capable of verification. They exclude assertive opinions, infused by emotions, desires or ideals. I wish also to express my gratitude to the following:

* My friend and colleague Dr. George Ramsden, for reading the manuscript, effecting corrections and offering useful suggestions.

* Mrs Ruth Kirkham, National Tutor Trainer of The Keep Fit Association, for the Foreword, contribution to chapter 8 and demonstration of skilful movements, to which drawings of stills cannot do justice. She has also offered helpful comments.

* CHURCHILL LIVINGSTONE (Longman Group) of Edinburgh— London—New York, for permission to reproduce illustrations from the popular McNAUGHT & CALLANDER : ILLUSTRATED PHYSIOLOGY, a wealth of anatomical and physiological lucid information.

* THE NATIONAL FILM BOARD OF CANADA, for permission to use stills for the front and back cover of this book, from Norman McLaren's famous PAS DE DEUX film.

* My dear wife, Irene, for painstakingly reading the proofs, her tolerance and secretarial assistance. She is the Training Secretary of The Keep Fit Association—South West Region.

B.H. Barrada

MB., Ch.B., M.R.C.S.(Eng.), L.R.C.P.(Lond.)

INTRODUCTION

This book is a physical fitness guide expressly written for those who desire to be, and stay fit. Its scope is necessarily limited in the interests of brevity; the aim has been to combine simplicity and clarity with accuracy.

To avoid confusion, only the relevant information needed to guide the reader in understanding and, it is hoped, enhancing his (her) physical strength and stamina, is given.

So much of our mind and conduct is influenced by the state of our body, and it is the mind which creates the world about us. Competence and readiness are required to equip us for the world's tasks.

Knowledge of fitness should be based on sense-recognised facts. This means acquaintance with (i) the form of the various structures which make up the human being: the shape and fabric of the body's parts, their arrangement and inter-relationship; (ii) the forces acting on the body and the motions effected by them; (iii) the vital processes of the body and their purpose. In short, body **structure**, **mechanics** and **functions**.

Let 'FITNESS FIRST' keep you fit.

Order of the book

1

Chapter 1

WHAT IS FITNESS, ITS PURPOSE AND VALUE?

The succeeding chapters are concerned with the two principal agencies which keep us fit: **movement** and **diet** or regulated and regular exercise and nutrition. These determine the state of our circulation, metabolism and drainage of waste-products — the pillars upon which the quality of life relies.

Health and fitness

Health and fitness share the characteristic of well-being in which all functions of the body are regularly performed. A child may be healthy but not fit or suitable for many tasks, physically or mentally, unable to adapt, either his body or mind, to the **environment** or the surrounding **influences** of the outside world.

Fitness is not an innate gift, endowed by nature, but an acquired state, the existence of which needs training, constancy and perseverance. To be fit is to possess strength, endurance and resilience.

The demarcation line between health and fitness is a distinct one, whereas health is absence of disease, fitness is a state of readiness to face and adapt ourselves to the environment and the surrounding influences, and at the same time experience the pleasure of well-being.

Definition of fitness

Fitness is the adaptability or adjustment of **body** and **mind** to render them better suited to face the world in our struggle for survival. Its basic constituent elements are: (a) **strength** (the foundation), which means the ability to exert pressure and withstand stress; (b) **stamina** or the power of endurance — a time factor; (c) **flexibility** (resilience or suppleness), involving a wide range of mobility.

5

The acquisition of fitness needs effort, "Restfulness is a quality for cattle; the virtues are all active, life is alert".

Two groups of systems

Our body has two groups of systems, arranged in accordance with our awareness of them. Willingness and determination are required to **adapt** them to the environment.

Group 1 This group of systems governs the continual chemical changes in the living body which take place during circulation, respiration, digestion, secretion, excretion, growth, repair and regeneration. Many of the activities of this group go on **below** the level of consciousness. The systems themselves are usually termed the "vegetative systems", so called since they function involuntarily and automatically like vegetation or plant life. Their regulation in the human body is mainly through the **Autonomic** Nervous System.

Group 2 This group of systems admits our **control** over the way the body reacts to the environment. It consists of two anatomical systems: the collective **Nervous System** and the Skeletal **Muscular** System. These are the commanding systems.

The aim

The aim of the entire exposition, disclosed in this booklet, is to resolve the process of **physical** fitness* which are regular and

---

* Mental fitness is the concern of another book entitled, the **HUMAN COMPUTER** — the Power of Effective Communication, which means eloquence by a short route — **ideas** and **words** to express them — a verbal encyclopaedia: showing how to organise thoughts and clothe them with apt words for every occasion of speaking or writing, in whatever walk of life.

The book can benefit all, be he or she a lover, student, tradesman, social worker, trade unionist, candidate, politician, journalist, author or a member of any of the professions. It will provide the reader with a flexible and well-furnished mind, and a heightened sense of power and self-confidence which springs from the knowledge that, whatever the situation, he (she) has the **mental** and **verbal** resources to control it.

The book provides **actual words** to be used for all occasions when spoken or written words are called for. The topics treated in the order of their appearance are: Instant Practical Steps, **Memory**, Particular Expressions, **Voice**, **Humour**, Entertainment, Repartee, **Love**, Art of **Persuasion**, **Discourse**: Description, Discussion, Explanation, regulated exercise and nutrition. It is not only to lay bare the premise upon which **movement** and **diet** are based, but to reveal the parts of which they consist and their interrelatedness and the steps by which fitness is derived from them.

Our first wealth is fitness in health.

The foundation of all knowledge

Since the ability to memorise is the foundation of all knowledge, every attempt is made to present the subject of **fitness** with **meaning** and **order**. Experience without meaning or order cannot be remembered for long. The more intense the meaning or order of an experience, the sharper and easier will be the recall. It is well to recall that any new knowledge, whether of bodily or mental habits is initially tediously acquired, but is rendered less strenuous by practice and repetition until the whole activity becomes almost automatic. The method adopted throughout these pages is that of coherent analysis of body structure and functions.

The ensuing chapters, therefore, have followed a definite plan in the expectation of securing your attention, based on interest, as the foundation of your memorising. Your assimilation is reinforced by the visual imagery of the illustrations. These will serve as supplementary to 'organisation' or the logical grouping together of common qualities. Your final consolidation, of course, can be achieved by repetition.

Now for chapter 2 and 'NATURE OF MOVEMENT': hold-the-door!

Exposition, Narrative, Correspondence, Interview, Proposition, Agreement, Analysis, Summary, Report and Paraphrase. The method of how to frame your thoughts and express them in apt words is revealed.

"It is what we **think we know already** that often prevents us from learning".

Chapter 2

THE NATURE OF MOVEMENT

If there is spontaneous movement there is life. This is the verdict of nature. Rest! You have all eternity to rest in.

Movement is the alteration or variation of position.

In our development from a fertilised cell to a multicellular creature, aggregates of cells have differentiated themselves to furnish highly specialised functions. The cells are arranged to provide a structural and functional fabric or texture, termed **tissue**. Tissues are grouped into sets of connected parts, termed **systems**.

Movement is carried out by the **Locomotor** System (muscles and bones) under the control of the Nervous System. The locomotor system embraces (a) the **skeleton** and (b) the skeletal **musculature**, skeletal so called because of its attachment to the skeleton. The rest of the body's musculature provides movement to and is embodied in the viscera, which are the internal organs, mainly the heart, blood vessels and bowels. These possess different muscular tissues from those of the skeletal muscles, and are **innervated** (nerve activated) **below** the level of consciousness.

The human skeleton — a structural base

The skeletal system is the rigid framework (mainly of calcium phosphate) of the body and consists of bones and joints. Its construction confers, not only movement but shape (build or figure) and attachment to muscles, and protection for the internal delicate organs.

Three distinctive varieties of bone

Bones may be classified according to their shape: (1) Flat. (2) Long. (3) Short. These are in addition to a large unclassified group.

9

See illustration, figure 1

(1) The flat bones of the skull, breast (sternum) and iliacs of the pelvis. These protect soft organs.

(2) The **long** bones of the arms (humerus, ulna and radius), and the legs (femur, tibia and fibula). These act as **levers** (rigid bars) able to move **at** a joint **about** a stationary **axis**. The axis itself is the pivot or **fulcrum** about which a lever turns.

(3) The **short** bones of the wrists and ankles. These afford united strength and extra mobility.

(4) Other lesser classified bones include: (a) The **ribs** which protect the heart and lungs; the **clavicles** (collar bones); the **scapulae** (shoulder blades). (b) The **vertebral** column, which provides a basis for the skeleton, forms a hollow canal protecting the spinal cord. The vertebral column comprises 33 vertebrae: **7** cervical, **12** thoracic, **5** lumbar, **5** fused sacral forming a thick curved bone, termed the **sacrum**, and **4** tail bones, termed **coccyx**. (c) Two **pubic** (in front) and two **ischial** (beneath) bones, fused with the flat iliac bones to form the pelvic girdle or **pelvis**. The pubis in front and the ischium in the rear. The ischium refers, of course, to the two ischial bones which bear the weight of the trunk in the sitting position. (d) The **patella** or knee-cap is the rounded bone protecting the knee joint. The **calcaneum** is the foot rear bone or heel bone. It bears most of our weight whilst standing and is raised with every step we take by the calf muscles. The rest of the weight is borne by the heads of the five **metatarsals**, which are the small long bones of the foot, forming a transverse arch. There are, of course, a series of transverse arches behind the heads of the metatarsals and two longitudinal arches: the inside which is flexible and the outside which is firm.

The joints

Joints are the place of union or articulation of bones. For the sake of clarity, brevity and ease of description, they are classified according to their degree of mobility into three classes:

(1) **Fixed** joints with no real ability to move, as between the bones of the skull. In fact the existence of the serrated sutures resists movement.

LOCOMOTOR SYSTEM

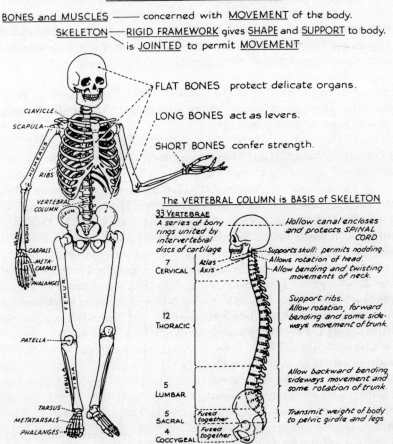

BONES and MUSCLES ——— concerned with MOVEMENT of the body.

SKELETON — RIGID FRAMEWORK gives SHAPE and SUPPORT to body.
is JOINTED to permit MOVEMENT

FLAT BONES protect delicate organs.

LONG BONES act as levers.

SHORT BONES confer strength.

CLAVICLE
SCAPULA
HUMERUS
RIBS
VERTEBRAL COLUMN
ILEUM
ULNA
RADIUS
CARPALS
META-CARPALS
PHALANGES
FEMUR
PATELLA
FIBULA
TIBIA
TARSUS
METATARSALS
PHALANGES

The VERTEBRAL COLUMN is BASIS of SKELETON

33 VERTEBRAE
A series of bony rings united by intervertebral discs of cartilage

7 CERVICAL — Atlas, Axis

12 THORACIC

5 LUMBAR

5 SACRAL — Fused together

4 COCCYGEAL — Fused together

Hollow canal encloses and protects SPINAL CORD
Supports skull: permits nodding.
Allows rotation of head.
Allow bending and twisting movements of neck.

Support ribs.
Allow rotation, forward bending and some sideways movement of trunk.

Allow backward bending, sideways movement and some rotation of trunk.

Transmit weight of body to pelvic girdle and legs.

All bones give attachment to muscles.

Figure 1

(2) **Semi-movable** where movement is not possible to any remarkable extent, where the bony surfaces are joined by a strong elastic fibro-cartilage (gristle). Such joints exist between the vertebrae. In the neck they collectively allow rotation of the head, as well as bending and stretching movement of the neck. In the trunk they permit backward stretching, forward bending, sideways movement and some rotation when twisting the trunk. Between the bones of the wrist and ankle some gliding movement takes place.

(3) **Movable joints**. These are classified according to their **range** of mobility. They all possess similar structure of ligamentous (tough bands) capsule and lubricating fluid. There are 3 main types: (i) **pivot**; (ii) **hinge**; (iii) **freely movable**.

(i) The **pivot** joints as exist between the two bones of the forearm which allow their rotation: (a) The upper **radio-ulnar** joint (see diagram, fig. 2), just below the elbow joint. This forms a pivot joint between the circumference of the rounded head of the **radius** and the smooth notch of the **ulna**; (b) The lower **radio-ulnar** joint, just above the wrist joint. This forms a pivot joint formed between the lower end of the **radius** and an ulnar notch. The word **pivot** simply means a centre on which anything turns. Movement is more pronounced at the upper (proximal) radio-ulnar joint than the lower (distal) joint. The movements at these two joints are those of **pronation** and **supination**. Pronation means rotating the forearm in such a way that the palm of the hand ends by looking downwards. **Supination** is the reverse movement: to turn the forearm and the hand so the palm looks upwards. The words

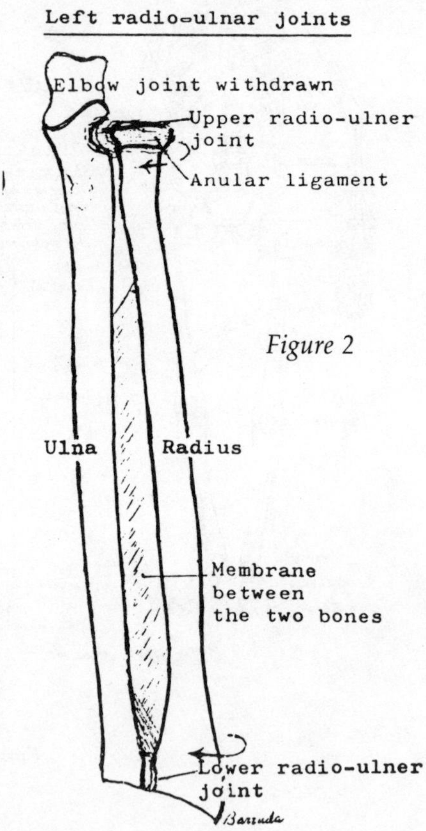

Left radio-ulnar joints

Elbow joint withdrawn

Upper radio-ulner joint

Anular ligament

Figure 2

Ulna   Radius

Membrane between the two bones

Lower radio-ulner joint

Barruda

12

pronation and supination come from the prone position, lying face downward, and the supine, lying on the back. The upper or **proximal radio-ulnar** is supported by a strong ligamentous capsule (anular ring) containing, of course, lubricating fluid.

(ii) The **hinge** joints, moving about an axis as in the **elbow** and **knee**. The axis of each joint lies horizontally in the erect standing position of the body with the palm of the hands facing forward (the body's anatomical position). Like any moveable joint, they are supported by a tough capsule and containing lubricating fluid.

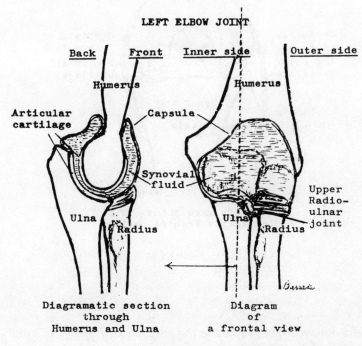

LEFT ELBOW JOINT

Back   Front   Inner side   Outer side

Humerus   Humerus

Articular cartilage

Capsule

Synovial fluid

Upper Radio-ulnar joint

Ulna   Ulna

Radius   Radius

Diagramatic section through Humerus and Ulna

Diagram of a frontal view

Figure 3

The **elbow** joint (see diagram, fig. 3) is a true **hinge** joint formed by ends of the bones of the upper arm and forearm: (a) the **humerus**, a single bone of the upper arm, and (b) the **ulna** and **radius** of the forearm. The articulating surfaces of the three bones are covered with a smooth elastic cartilage (gristle). The upper ends of the ulna and radius together form a cup-shaped articulating surface into which the rounded end of the humerus appropriately fits. The hinge movement allows full flexion but no hyperextension. The ulnar bone is the most exposed part of the elbow and is easily damaged. The elbow joint is supported by a capsule, lined with a synovial membrane, which secretes a clear lubricating fluid.

The **knee** joint (see diagram, fig.4) is a **hinge** joint formed by the two-knobbed lower end of the femur (thigh bone) and the gently-hollowed upper end of the tibia (shin bone). The inner surface of the

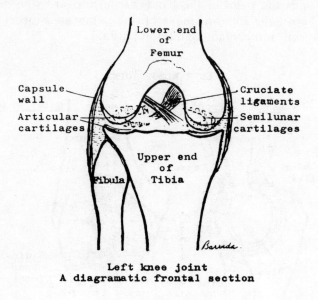

Left knee joint
A diagramatic frontal section

Figure 4

patella (knee-cap) is adapted to the articular surface of the femur. All three articulating surfaces are covered with a smooth elastic cartilage. In addition there are two intervening gristle pads, termed **semilunar** cartilages; if either is injured, full extension is prevented by a locking mechanism. Two considerably stronger ligaments cross each other in the middle of the joint: these are the **cruciate** ligaments. Further extension of the knee is prevented by the tenseness of these cruciate ligaments and, of course, by the firm binding of the ligamentous capsule and the surrounding muscles. Apart from the hinge movement of extension and flexion, the knee is capable of a limited rotation either way, which renders the knee joint not a true hinge joint. The

14

capsule of the knee joint is lined with a synovial membrane which secretes a clear lubricating fluid.

(iii) The **freely movable** joints have a **ball-and-socket** construction. They are capable of considerable movement: extension, flexion, abduction (away from the body's middle line), adduction (towards the middle line), and rotation (revolving round an axis, outward or inward). A ligamentous capsule envelops the joint, lined with a synovial membrane which secretes a clear lubricating fluid.

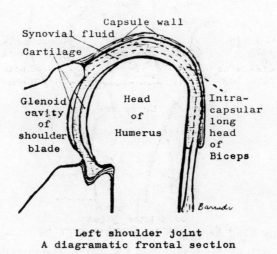

Left shoulder joint
A diagramatic frontal section

Figure 5

The **shoulder** joint (see diagram, fig.5) is formed by the large hemispherical head of the humerus and the small shallow cup-shaped outer-angled head-like lump of the triangle-shaped shoulder-blade (scapula). The articular surfaces are covered with elastic fibro-cartilage. The joint's strength is largely dependent on the support of the surrounding muscles. Because of the shallow articular cavity, termed the glenoid, laxity of the capsule and freedom of movement, the joint is easily dislocated. In a dislocation, the head of humerus could tear through the capsule. It is treated by manipulation under anaesthesia.

15

The **hip** joint (see diagram, fig.6) is a ball-and-socket joint. It is the strongest and largest joint in the body. It supports the weight of the trunk, with the head, neck and arms. It is formed by the large head of

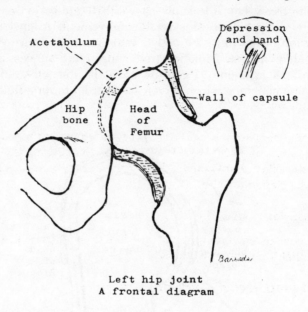

Left hip joint
A frontal diagram

Figure 6

the femur, the longest bone, and the deep cup-shaped cavity (acetabulum) of the hip bone of the pelvis. The articulating surfaces are covered with cartilage. A flattened band of strong fibrous tissue extends from a depression in the head of the femur to a notch in the cavity rim (acetabular notch). The femur's neck may be rarefied with age and is a common site of fracture.

Flexibility of joints

Flexibility of a joint is the **extent** within which a joint can operate effectively — its amplitude, limit or range.

To prepare, adapt and adjust your body to life's physical tasks (fitness), you need **enduring strength**, not only of the muscles acting on the joint, but also of every part of a joint. These parts consist of: cartilage; synovial membrane lining the capsule (shell, case or bag) which secretes the lubricating fluid; ligaments, whether internal or external to the capsule.

Resistance or interference to movement restrains or narrows the *range of mobility*, i.e., flexibility. Such restraint occurs in **injury** (torn cartilage, capsule or ligament) or in **disease** such as inflamed synovial membrane or arthritis. It must be emphasised that weakness, injury or disease of the **muscles** acting on a joint, take precedence in our reckoning of flexibility. Further, hyper-mobility, as in some sports, may lead to a joint's temporary or permanent instability. It is well to realise that articular cartilages have no sensation (no nerve supply), but should they weaken, waste or calcify as occurs in unfit old age, pain develops through affecting the surrounding parts.

Complete natural flexibility with a wide range of mobility, through active muscular self-exertion, is termed **dynamic** flexibility. Achieving flexibility with outside help (passive movement), however, is termed **static** flexibility.

Conclusion

The conclusion to which we are led then, is that flexibility is an essential ingredient of fitness.

Test your recognising powers

Give a distinctive name, meaningful title or caption by which the movement or its range can be identified in the proceeding figures.

If you can score 12 out of 23 you will have the satisfaction of knowing that you have accomplished the first stage in the mastery of the subject! Full list of titles appear on the page following the figures.

The next chapter will deal with what from the reader's viewpoint is the most important item in the nature of movement, namely, contractility or muscular action. This will involve group action of muscles and their co-ordination.

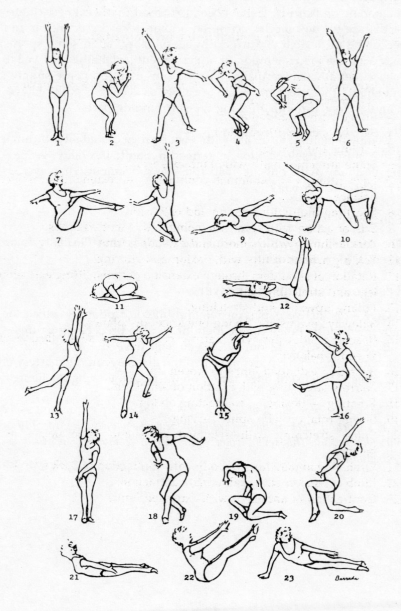

Figure 7

18

A WIDE RANGE OF MOBILITY

Giving a name, title or caption to the preceding figures

1. Spine stretching and arm extension reaching high.
2. Contraction of abdomen and flexion of joints to maximise abdominal contraction.
3. Lunge with extended arms.
4. Sideways curl with rotation.
5. Curling and flexing.
6. Spine stretching with wide limb extension.
7. Legs lifting — abdominal contraction — extended arms for balance.
8. Reaching high with rotation and extension.
9. Scissor action with spine stretching and extended limbs.
10. Back arching with rotation, and extended arms.
11. Folding around centre with flexion and curving.
12. Rotation of shoulders through extension of arms, lifting extended legs and stretching spine.
13. Pulling upwards and stretching.
14. Sideways extension, flexing one knee for balance.
15. Reaching sideways with narrow curving and slight flexion of knee for balance.
16. Swinging extended limbs to loosen up.
17. Narrow stretching with rotation of shoulders.
18. Rotating — flexing — contracting abdomen.
19. Strong rotation with spine curving.
20. Spine stretching with extended arms and knee flexion for balance.
21. Stretching and arching of body with contraction of back muscles.
22. Limb extension with abdominal contraction.
23. Contraction of abdomen with extended limbs.

Chapter 3

CONTRACTILITY — THE POWER BEHIND THE MOVEMENT

Group action of muscles: co-ordination

Muscles by nature are assembled in groups. They work in co-operation with each other, not in isolation, whatever the movement. This integrated activity is for the purpose of effective movement. The function of members of the group is identified by name as follows:

(1) **Prime movers**. These are the leaders of the contesting movement, termed **agonists**, or more appropriately, **protagonists**. Examples:

Flexion at the elbow joint, a hinge joint (see illustration of Muscular Movements, fig. 8) The lever is the forearm. The fulcrum (in the anatomical position) is the horizontal axis, centrally placed in the joint, about which the forearm turns in an upward direction to bring it closer to the upper arm (flexion). This means pulling the forearm towards the upper arm. The pulling force is produced by the contraction of the brachialis and biceps muscles, applied at their respective insertions to the ulna and radius (bones of the forearm). The brachialis and biceps muscles are the prime movers.

The manner of a prime mover's contraction is to **shorten** its own length, by increasing the internal muscular tension, which is the pulling force.

Flexion at the knee joint, a hinge joint (see illustration of Skeletal muscles — back view, fig. 10). The prime movers are the hamstring muscles of the back of the thigh. They pull the lower leg towards the thigh at the knee joint.

(2) **Antagonists**. These produce an opposite action to the prime movers in their effort of co-ordination, i.e., integration in a harmonious

MUSCULAR MOVEMENTS

The long bones particularly form a light framework of LEVERS.
The skeletal muscles attached to them contract to operate these levers.

When a muscle contracts it shortens.

This brings its two ends closer together.

Since the two ends are attached to different bones by TENDONS one or other of the bones must move.

Two bones meet or articulate at a JOINT.

Joint surfaces are covered with a layer of smooth CARTILAGE.

To avoid friction when the two surfaces move on one another a SYNOVIAL MEMBRANE secretes a
                                    LUBRICATING FLUID.

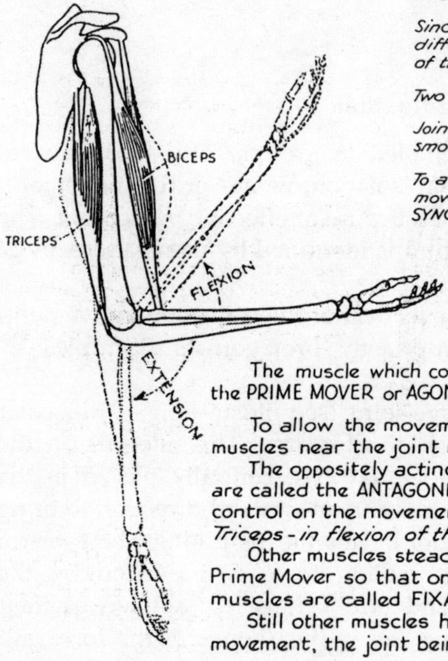

BICEPS

TRICEPS

FLEXION

EXTENSION

The muscle which contracts to move the joint is called the PRIME MOVER or AGONIST *(the Biceps in flexion of elbow)*

To allow the movement to take place, however, other muscles near the joint must co-operate :-
The oppositely acting muscles gradually relax – these are called the ANTAGONISTS and exercise a "braking" control on the movement. *(e.g. the EXTENSORS – chiefly Triceps - in flexion of the elbow.)*

Other muscles steady the bone giving "origin" to the Prime Mover so that only the "insertion" will move – these muscles are called FIXATORS.

Still other muscles help to steady, for most efficient movement, the joint being moved — called SYNERGISTS.

When the elbow is straightened the reverse occurs:-
TRICEPS, the Prime Mover, CONTRACTS; BICEPS, the Antagonist, RELAXES.

Figure 8

SKELETAL MUSCLES

Bones are moved at joints by the CONTRACTION and RELAXATION of MUSCLES attached to them.

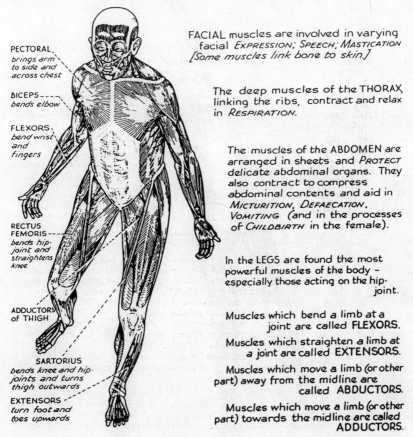

PECTORAL,
brings arm
to side and
across chest

BICEPS
bends elbow

FLEXORS,
bend wrist
and
fingers

RECTUS
FEMORIS
bends hip·
joint and
straightens
knee

ADDUCTORS
of THIGH

SARTORIUS
bends knee and hip·
joints and turns
thigh outwards

EXTENSORS
turn foot and
toes upwards

FACIAL muscles are involved in varying facial *EXPRESSION; SPEECH; MASTICATION* *[Some muscles link bone to skin.]*

The deep muscles of the THORAX, linking the ribs, contract and relax in *RESPIRATION.*

The muscles of the ABDOMEN are arranged in sheets and *PROTECT* delicate abdominal organs. They also contract to compress abdominal contents and aid in *MICTURITION, DEFAECATION, VOMITING* (and in the processes of *CHILDBIRTH* in the female).

In the LEGS are found the most powerful muscles of the body – especially those acting on the hip-joint.

Muscles which bend a limb at a joint are called FLEXORS.

Muscles which straighten a limb at a joint are called EXTENSORS.

Muscles which move a limb (or other part) away from the midline are called ABDUCTORS.

Muscles which move a limb (or other part) towards the midline are called ADDUCTORS.

Figure 9

23

SKELETAL MUSCLES

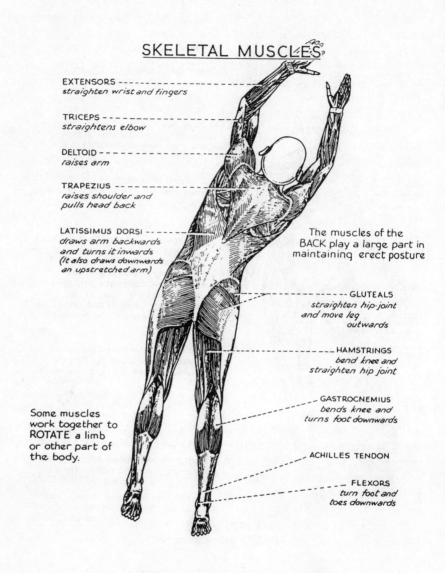

EXTENSORS ------------------
straighten wrist and fingers

TRICEPS ------------------
straightens elbow

DELTOID ------------------
raises arm

TRAPEZIUS --------------
*raises shoulder and
pulls head back*

LATISSIMUS DORSI --------
*draws arm backwards
and turns it inwards
(It also draws downwards
an upstretched arm)*

The muscles of the
BACK play a large part in
maintaining erect posture

----------- **GLUTEALS**
*straighten hip-joint
and move leg
outwards*

----------- **HAMSTRINGS**
*bend knee and
straighten hip joint*

GASTROCNEMIUS
*bends knee and
turns foot downwards*

Some muscles
work together to
ROTATE a limb
or other part of
the body.

ACHILLES TENDON

FLEXORS
*turn foot and
toes downwards*

Figure 10

24

operation. They often produce an opposite action to the prime movers (the protagonists). This means that when the prime movers contract, the antagonists relax and vice versa. They are governed by a *reciprocal innervation*, which is a mutual beneficial distribution of nerves. Thus any contraction of a prime mover is accompanied by relaxation of its antagonist to achieve co-ordination or harmony. One thing is certain: that they are eternally co-ordinators but not always antagonists. Should the intention, however, be to keep a joint unmoved, the prime movers and antagonists would *contract simultaneously*, e.g., the biceps and triceps both contract together to keep the elbow fixed as when attempting to punch with a clenched fist (try this now to prove it to yourself). The simultaneous contractions continue with the movement of the arm to deliver the punch. Similarly, when attempting a stroke at golf with the extended arms, the biceps or triceps act as prime movers, acting simultaneously in co-ordination. Muscles in health will always be in functional harmony to achieve the desired position or movement.

The **cerebellum**, the round nerve-tissue mass at the back and base of the head, discharges impulses which give, not only *co-ordination* of muscles, but also a sense of *balance*.

(3) **Fixators**. These muscles co-operate to firm and stabilise the bones giving origin to prime movers, for *functional effectiveness*. Example: Flexion at the elbow joint. The forearm is pulled by the contraction of the brachialis and biceps (the prime movers) towards the upper arm. The brachialis originates from the humerus (bone of the upper arm) and biceps from the outer angle of the shoulder blade (scapula). Both their insertion is the forearm (the lever). Some of the muscles of the upper arm and shoulder act as **fixators** for the prime movers effectively to pull the forearm in the direction of the shoulder, which is flexion at the elbow joint.

Thus fixators fix the bones supplying the muscles origin to facilitate the movement initiated by the prime movers.

(4) **Synergists**. These work with the prime movers to *control and direct the movement*. Unlike the antagonists and fixators, their function is to modify or alter the direction of the pull of prime movers to the most advantageous position. Their action is better understood when the tendons (ligament, band or cord) of prime movers pass over more than one joint. Examples: (a) In holding a club with the thicker end

uppermost, the fingers are flexed to hold the narrow end with the exception of the extended forefinger, to direct the hold or movement of the club. (b) In making a stroke with a brush when painting a picture, the extended thumb, fore and middle fingers direct the movement of the brush whilst the two little fingers are flexed (not unlike writing). (c) In any stick or bat used to strike a ball in various sports, the fingers hold the stick and direct the movement to the most advantageous position. The prime movers in all these examples are the flexors and/or extensors of the fingers whose origin is the forearm. The long tendons pass over the wrist and the small joints of the hand to reach the fingers. The **synergists** are the short and intermediate muscles of the hand, including the lumricals and interossei which direct, modify or alter the initial action of the prime movers. The synergists give the movement a greater precision.

Having dealt with the systems and parts working together to produce body movement, there remains the forces acting on the body and the motions produced by them, i.e., **body mechanics***, which will be the subject of the succeeding chapter.*

Chapter 4

BODY MECHANICS

The task of knowing body mechanics with comprehension, so fearful and formidable a subject to most people, can in reality be quite simple. These pages are intended to unfold the principles of the gravitational force, its centre, line and base; equilibrium or balance; mechanics of movement, the direction of pull, effect of speed, the motion's quantity or momentum.

All muscle cells which serve various systems possess the power to contract. Active conscious movement exercises are the great foundation of fitness. The skeletal or voluntary **muscles** operate the rigid bars of **bone** (levers) which stir and propel the body.

Mechanics of position

The mechanical principles which should be borne in mind when considering body position or posture are the following:

(1) The principle of **gravity**. This is a continually acting force by which the human body is attracted downward to the earth. If this gravitational force is not opposed by the body's static muscular contractility (muscle firmness, termed **tone**), then the body falls to the ground. To maintain the body in any position, static or active, an **opposing** internal force, produced by muscular contraction (tension), is needed. Such a force must, at least, be equal to the gravitational force occasioned by the body weight.

(2) The **centre** of the gravitational force, in the standing erect position is in the sacrum, about the 2nd sacral vertebra or higher depending on height. The sacrum, it will be recalled is a thick curved bone, formed by the fusion of 5 sacral bones at the lower end of the back, holding the two halves of the pelvis together (see illustration, fig. 11).

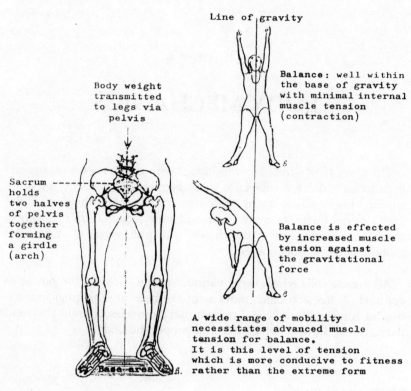

Line of gravity

Body weight
transmitted
to legs via
pelvis

Balance: well within
the base of gravity
with minimal internal
muscle tension
(contraction)

Sacrum
holds
two halves
of pelvis
together
forming
a girdle
(arch)

Balance is effected
by increased muscle
tension against
the gravitational
force

Base area

A wide range of mobility
necessitates advanced muscle
tension for balance.
It is this level .of tension
which is more conducive to fitness
rather than the extreme form

Figure 11

The gravitational weight-force of the upper part of the body consisting of trunk, head and neck, and arms, is transmitted from the **sacrum** to the head of the **femur**. Theoretically, such a force is shaped as an arch (see illustration, fig. 11). The gravitational force is then transmitted, at each side, to the femur, then through the legs to the feet.

Experiment: try now to raise your heels from the ground whilst standing, you will feel the contraction of the calf muscles. This strong contraction-force would oppose and exceed the gravitational force, enabling you to raise your heels. The contracting calf muscles are the paunchy **gastrocnemius** (Greek gaster = belly), in front of which is the broad **soleus**. Both possess considerable power. The gastrocnemius (fig. 10) is the propelling force in walking, running and leaping. The soleus is the leg's steadying force in the standing position. The sole of the foot is extended (straightened) when the heel

28

is raised. When the heel moves up it distances itself from the ball of the foot.

(3) The effective **base** of gravity: The centre of gravity of a solid geometric cube, having equally identical sides, will be its middle point. Its **line** of gravity will be its vertical axis. But the real effective and operative gravitational force occasioned by its weight will be acting on its base, namely the square area touching the ground.

Similarly the **line** of a human body's gravitational force, in the erect standing position, is a vertical line extending from the centre of the head through the centre of the sacrum to a central point between the feet. The effective gravitational **base**, of course, is the contacting area which supports the feet and between the feet, termed the base area (fig. 11). If all parts of the body are uniformly within the base, a state of **equilibrium** or balance then exists, just as with a horizontal rod balanced at a point (fulcrum) exactly half-way along its length. If the body bends, the line of gravity changes towards the more weighty part and consequent imbalance. Similarly, if you hold a weight in your hand with an outstretched arm, the line of gravity will move towards the weight and could be outside the base, depending on the gravitational force of that weight.

To sum up: the two forces working in opposition are the external force of **gravity** and the internal force of muscular **contractility**. Stability exists when the forces are fully balanced and within the margins of the gravitational **base**.

The healthy posture

The reason why many people have forwardly dropped-head, arched-shoulders, humped-back, often developed in later life, is that most of our daily activities are carried out by the muscles of the front and not those of the back, which latter become weaker and weaker with consequent imbalance. Daily morning stretching exercises to support an erect figure, the habit of standing tall with expanded oxygen-intaking chest, and abdomen drawn in with occasional abdominal muscular contractions — all these will ensure a healthy posture.

Mechanics of movement

If the tension force of muscular contraction equals the force of gravity, no movement takes place as in the erect standing-still position already explained. Also, unmodified straight downward movement of a raised arm needs only the force of gravity. An upward movement, on the other hand, is only effected by the internal muscular contraction force **exceeding** and **opposing** the force of gravity.

Direction of pull

Long bones in the body represent rigid bars (**levers**), capable of movement about a fixed point or axis, termed **fulcrum**. The articulated surfaces of a joint determine and symbolise the fulcrum. Although movements of the body occur at joints, nonetheless a joint is the point of support of a lever and the type and range of movement is influenced by the articulating surfaces of a joint (see chapter 2). Movement takes place in the **plane** which lies at right angles to the axis, not unlike the hands of a clock moving round the central pin or axis over the clock face, which is at right angles to the pin (the axis).

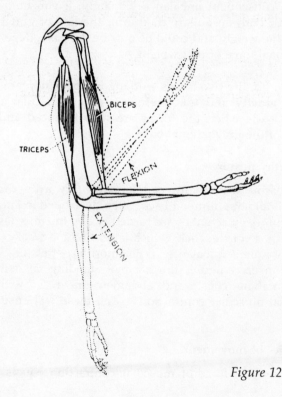

Figure 12

30

The less movable of the two areas of attachment of a muscle is its **origin**, usually a stable part of the skeleton. The attachment to a more mobile part of bone is termed the **insertion**. The **direction** of movement is determined by the position of the insertion to the bone. The latter is pulled towards the muscle origin (see illustration, fig. 12). The pull is most effective if the muscle is inserted at right angles to the bone; the effectiveness decreases as the angle of pull diminishes. Direction of movement, of course, is governed by all the operative forces producing the movement, supremely amongst them is that of the brain.

Effect of speed

Initial rapid movement requires added internal muscular tension (force), but when a **momentum** (the motion's quantity) is gathered, lesser contraction-tension is necessary to maintain the movement. This is not unlike the free-wheeling of a car after gathering speed-momentum, which is an increasing force derived from its motion. Momentum is the product of the mass and its velocity, for any motion in a straight line, i.e., Momentum = Mass × Velocity (speed or rapidity).

The next chapter will deal with the equally important subject of muscular **energy** — *this dynamic power, both at rest and during exercise, and its source. It will also treat muscle* **tone** *and muscle* **fatigue**.

Chapter 5

ENERGY — A DYNAMIC POWER

Energy produced in the body is an accumulated power available for use physically and mentally. It can be determined physically in terms of work done, e.g., muscular energy measured in terms of lifting, say, 1 kilogram 100 cm high in 1 second. Energy is required also for the various bodily functions and in the young for fresh tissue formation.

The source of human energy is nutrition, which is the intake of food (protein, fat, carbohydrate, minerals, vitamins and water) and oxygen. Instant muscular energy is derived from carbohydrate and fat, mainly the former.

The average principal constituents of skeletal muscles are: water 80%; **protein** 17%; fat 0.2%; carbohydrate in the form of glycogen (human starch) 0.7+%; glucose in the blood capillaries 0.1%; minerals (mainly phosphates) together with vitamins and hormones 1%.

The end-product of carbohydrate digestion is glucose. This is absorbed into the blood stream. The resting blood glucose level is about 100 mgm of glucose per 100 c.c. of blood (0.1%), whereas blood cholesterol level (the human body synthesises cholesterol) is about 10–20 mgm per 100 c.c. (0.01% – 0.02%). Cholesterol is derived, in man, mainly from absorbed fatty acids and glycerine, the products of fat digestion. Glucose supplies the energy which allows the protein to build up cells for growth, repair and regeneration.

How muscular energy is created

Glucose ($C_6H_{12}O_6$) is oxidised in tissue cells by the oxygen carried by the oxyhaemoglobin of the blood from the lungs. The oxidation or combustion produces $CO_2 + H_2O$ + heat + energy. This is a chemical energy, necessary for all living cells in the body, and in the muscles it is converted into mechanical energy, not unlike the combustion of fuel-oil to produce mechanical power. This dynamic power is used to maintain muscle tone and elementary movements. In the presence of oxygen sufficiency, muscle glycogen is converted to CO_2 + H_2O + heat + energy, during muscular movement.

During vigorous muscular exercise and in the absence of sufficient oxygen, dependent on the severity and speed of exercise, muscle glycogen is converted anaerobically to **lactic acid**. The lactic acid circulates in the alkaline blood stream to become **lactate**, subsequently oxidised, often elsewhere, such as in the liver and heart. Some may even change back into glycogen.

The source of muscular energy thus is the **glycogen** in the muscles and the more muscular storage of glycogen the greater the **stamina** (power of endurance). Protein provides the strength.

Muscle tone

Muscle tone means muscle firmness or tautness and is a normal functioning of other organs. Firmness gives muscles their shape. Muscle tone diminishes with age and contours lessen as tone abates.

Muscular fatigue

Muscular fatigue is caused not only by oxygen lack but also by the accumulation of waste products of metabolism (the chemical changes in the tissues) and other toxins such as alcohol or drugs. Muscles are refreshed by any improved oxygenation (aerobic), flow of circulation, accelerated metabolism, drainage of tissue waste-products, through the agency of aerobic fitness exercises (regulated and regular).

To **sum up**, energy is the power of doing work. Stored glycogen in the muscles is the prime source of energy. It is the progressively trained muscles which afford expansion of muscle fibres with protein and greater storage capacity of glycogen — the foundation of muscular energy. As will be shown later, excess carbohydrate intake, by itself, will be converted into fat (adipose tissue).

The subject of 'musculature' cannot be complete without ascertaining the types of material or the various **muscular tissues** *which exist in the body. This will be the concern of the next chapter.*

Chapter 6

THE THREE VARIETIES OF MUSCULAR TISSUE

Characteristics of muscle cells

Muscle cells are elongated cells (units) having the power of **contractility**: the ability to contract, becoming smaller. This means the competence of pulling together their **protoplasmic** (living matter) content. The words 'protoplasm' and 'cytoplasm' are not uncommonly used as if interchangeable. See fig. 13.

They also have the ability to increase their length or relax with loss of driving power.

Muscular tissues

Tissues are collections of cells connected by their walls or other substance between them to form a texture, material or fabric. There are **three** distinguishable varieties of muscular tissue in the body. These are (fig. 14):

(1) **Smooth, unstriped involuntary** muscle tissue. This tissue is under the control of the **autonomic** (involuntary) nervous system, below the level of consciousness. This type of tissue exists in the walls of blood vessels and viscera (internal organs of body), sometimes creating contraction and relaxation, e.g., *peristalsis*, which is the slow wave-like contraction and relaxation of the alimentary canal (bowel).

(2) **Cardiac or heart muscle tissue**. The cells here are exceptionally highly specialised. Heart muscle cells have no regenerative power once destroyed. They can only be replaced by fibrous scar tissue.

Another supreme exception is the existence of a focus in the walls of the left auricle with the inherent ability of **initiating** and

DIFFERENTIATION of ANIMAL CELLS

SPECIALIZATION distinguishes multicellular creatures from more primitive forms of life.

ONE-CELLED ANIMALS Capable of INDEPENDENT existence —
Undifferentiated — Show all activities or ····PHENOMENA of LIFE

MANY-CELLED ANIMALS Cells CO-OPERATE for   *All cells retain powers of*
well-being of whole body.   *ORGANIZATION*
Differentiated —— Groups of cells undergo   *IRRITABILITY*
adaptations and sacrifice   *NUTRITION*
some powers to fit them   *METABOLISM*
for special duties.   *RESPIRATION*
EXCRETION

MODIFICATION   ····*for*   ··SPECIALIZATION   ··*with*·· LOSS or REDUCTION
of STRUCTURE···· *efficient*   of FUNCTION   of VERSATILITY
E.g.

SECRETORY CELL········ Highly developed powers   *Diminished powers of*
of SECRETION   CONTRACTION and
Cytoplasm   Nucleus   e.g. enzymes for   REPRODUCTION
displaced   chemical breakdown
to base by   of foodstuffs.
formed and
Nucleus····   stored
secretion

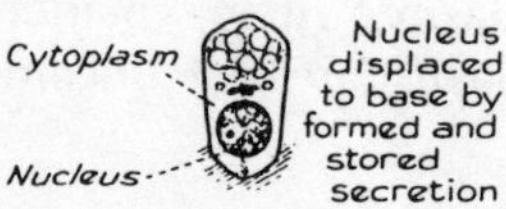

FAT CELL ················· STORAGE of FAT   *Loss of powers of*
Cytoplasm   CONTRACTION and
Cytoplasm   SECRETION
displaced
by stored
Nucleus   fat

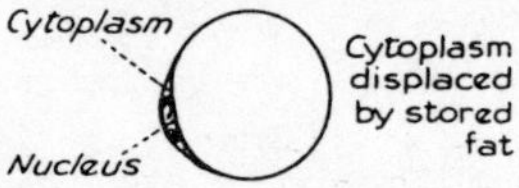

MUSCLE CELL············· Highly developed powers   *Diminished powers of*
of CONTRACTILITY   SECRETION and
Cytoplasm   Nucleus   REPRODUCTION

Elongated
cell body

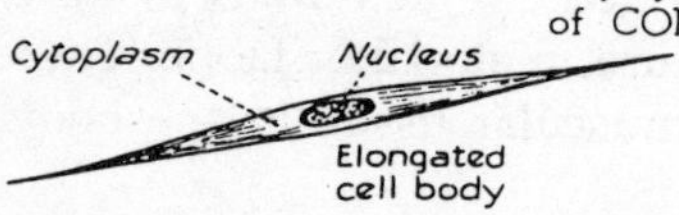

NERVE CELL············· Highly developed powers   *Loss of powers of*
Cytoplasm   of IRRITABILITY   REPRODUCTION

Cytoplasm   (response to stimuli   *ie. if nerve*
drawn out   and transmission of   *cell is destroyed*
Nucleus   into long   impulses over long   *no regeneration*
x500   branching   distances)   *is possible.*
processes

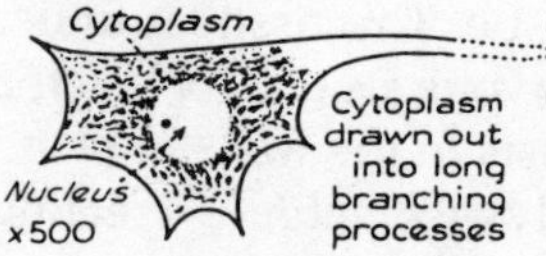

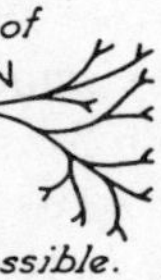

Figure 13

MUSCULAR TISSUES

All have ELONGATED cells with special development of CONTRACTILITY.

1. SMOOTH, UNSTRIPED, VISCERAL or INVOLUNTARY muscle

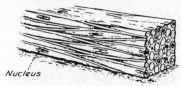

Nucleus

Least specialized.
Slow rhythmical contraction and relaxation.
Not under voluntary control.
Found in walls of viscera and blood vessels.

2. CARDIAC or HEART muscle

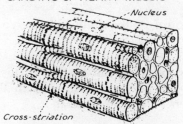

Nucleus

Cross-striation

More highly specialized.
Rapid rhythmical contraction (and relaxation) spreads through whole muscle mass.
Not under voluntary control.
Found only in heart wall.

3. STRIATED, STRIPED, SKELETAL or VOLUNTARY muscle

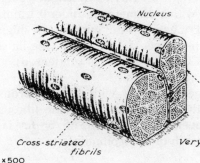

Nucleus

Thick covering membrane (sarcolemma)

Cross-striated fibrils

× 500

Most highly specialized.
Very rapid, powerful contractions of individual fibres.
Under voluntary control.
Found in e.g muscles of trunk, limbs, head.

Very long, large multi-nucleated units.
No branching.

Figure 14

maintaining rapid rhythmical muscular contraction of the heart. This node is the cardiac **pacemaker**. Its stimulus is transmitted through the heart at the rate of an average of 72 beats per minute. Duration of beat is thus about 0.8 second ($\frac{1}{72} \times 60$). These rhythmic contractions render the heart a driving **pump**.

Every time the contracting ventricles of the heart pump blood into the circulation, a wave of blood causes **expansion** of the elastic-walled arteries, termed **pulse**. This can readily be felt at the radial artery just above the wrist on the thumb-side, which gives an indication of the **rate** (frequency per minute) and **regularity** of the heart. Pulse rate is increased by emotion, exertion, fevers, endocrine (ductless glands) secretions, nervous or heart disorders, and certain drugs.

The heart is also under the control of the autonomic nervous system.

(3) **Striated, striped, skeletal**, termed **voluntary muscle tissue**. This is under voluntary control, by the brain and is concerned with the movement of the bony skeleton, hence the term **skeletal**.

The thin elongated cells are placed tightly together to form multi-nucleated muscle **fibres** or threads (fig. 15), varying in length from a fraction of a centimetre to 30 cms, with a **diameter** of under 0.1 mm. The individual fibres are bound together into bundles. A high magnification is required to see the stripes on the fibres (see illus-tration, but the MECHANISM of CONTRACTION is condensed).

Some muscle bundles converge to merge with tough fibrous tendons (ligaments) at one or both ends of a muscle. Thin fibrous tissue also forms a protective covering: muscle sheath or **fascia**. Voluntary muscle fibres do not branch or intercommunicate.

The bundles form the bulk of a skeletal muscle with channels between the bundles for the blood vessels and nerves which supply them. Skeletal muscles have attachments to the bony skeleton: origins and insertions. Some muscle tendons cross more than one joint before reaching their attachment to the bone.

In the interests of clarity and greater comprehension of fitness, a summary of body functions will be given in the remaining chapters. This will commence with the principal regulator and director of all other systems, the **Nervous**

System. *Its cells are intricately constructed and arranged to react to, integrate and conduct physical forces. It is the only system engaged in non-physical faculties of thought-feeling-intention (the mind) and recollection (the memory). It is truly the commanding system.*

SKELETAL MUSCLE
and the MECHANISM of CONTRACTION

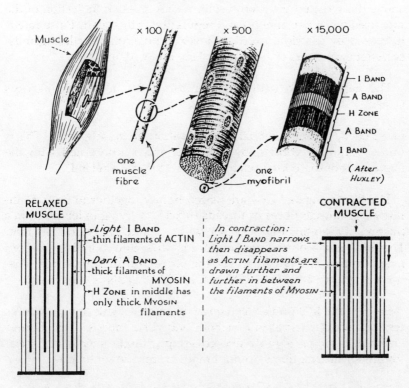

Muscle

x 100   x 500   x 15,000

I BAND
A BAND
H ZONE
A BAND
I BAND

(*After* HUXLEY)

one muscle fibre

one myofibril

RELAXED MUSCLE

Light I BAND
-thin filaments of ACTIN
Dark A BAND
-thick filaments of MYOSIN
H ZONE in middle has only thick MYOSIN filaments

In contraction:
Light I BAND narrows
then disappears
as ACTIN filaments are
drawn further and
further in between
the filaments of MYOSIN

CONTRACTED MUSCLE

Energy for contraction is derived from glucose and fat in the mitochondrion   The energy is transported from the mitochondrion to the contractile filaments in ATP. ATP splits readily into ADP and phosphate, releasing its trapped energy where needed.

Figure 15

Chapter 7

THE NERVOUS SYSTEM

Life's Satisfactions

We are all born with certain **instinctive urges** and **strivings** as well as bodily **appetites**. First in importance is the self-regarding instinct which expresses itself in a variety of ways, notably the **preservation of life** itself. This in turn — the preservation of life — involves bodily protection (shelter), securing food, maintenance of health (sleep and other bodily functions). These are all primitive necessities which must be satisfied if life is to continue, even at the lowest level.

At higher levels come the needs arising from the **growth** and **fulfilment of personality** including love (caring), companionship, religion (human values) and the development of individual powers of **mind** and **body**.

Except in the primitive forms of human society, the maintenance of these human relationships entails the acquisition of **property**, using the **term** in its widest sense to include possessions of every kind — inevitably the use of money, in whatever shape or form, as a medium of exchange, whether for immediate enjoyment or postponed enjoyment and greater present security, or both.

Mind and memory

Mind includes all conscious and subconscious experiences and their adjustment, which determines behaviour and manner of speech. Recalling the subconscious experiences into consciousness is **memory**.

The mind depends on the physical state of the **nerve cells** (neurons) which are a **material** agency, but what is mind? 'Never matter', 'What is matter?', 'Never mind'. This much is certain: 'Without body (matter) there can be no memory, and **without**

memory there can be no mind'. There is evidence produced by neuro-physiology experimenters that 'there is some structural change with memory'. Memory is not just a storing mechanism. 'If people stored all the nonsense they have seen they could never retrieve anything'. 'Molecules are constantly arranging new relationships'. There is evidence, however, of a magnetic field in the **frontal area of the brain** and the presence of an appreciable amount of iron in the vicinity.

Two groups of systems

Our **body** has two groups of systems, arranged in accordance with our awareness of them by the **mind**. Volition and determination, which are mental process, are needed to **adapt** them to the environment in our struggle for survival. This is **fitness**, which involves physical and mental agility, flexibility, balance, co-ordination, **stamina** and strength:

Group 1 The first group of systems admits our **control** over the way the body reacts to the environment, though not entirely. It consists of two anatomical systems: the **Nervous** System and the skeletal **Muscular** System.

Group 2 This group of systems governs the continual chemical changes in the living body which take place during circulation, respiration, digestion, secretion, excretion, growth, repair, regeneration and reproduction. Much of the activities of this group goes on **below the level of consciousness**. The systems themselves are usually termed the 'vegetative systems'. Their regulation is mainly through the **Autonomic** Nervous System (Greek autos = self, nomos = law), though partly and indirectly through the Central Nervous System which includes the brain. The anatomical term which embraces all these systems is simply the ***Nervous System***.

THE NERVOUS SYSTEM

The Nervous System embraces:

The brain and spinal cord, termed the Central Nervous System.
The issuing **nerves**, termed the Peripheral Nervous System.
The **Autonomic** Nervous System formed largely from a network of nerve cells and their fibres (in the chest and abdominal cavities),

termed the *Sympathetic* component and partly from cells arising from the hind part of the brain below the level of consciousness, termed the *Parasympathetic* component.

They all intercommunicate with each other.

The Central Nervous System: the **brain** and **spinal cord**.

The Brain(see diagram, fig. 16)

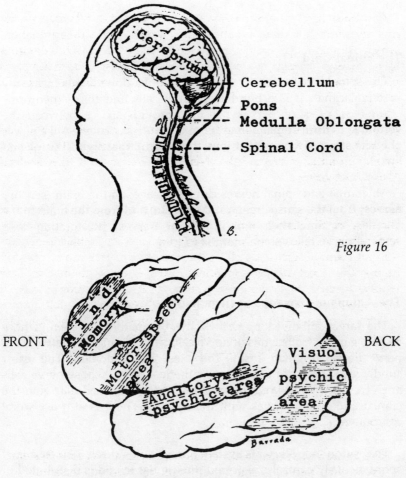

Cerebellum
Pons
Medulla Oblongata
Spinal Cord

Figure 16

FRONT   BACK

OUTER SURFACE OF LEFT HALF OF BRAIN
(CEREBRAL HEMISPHERE)

43

It is a soft mass with many folds within the skull (cranium), consisting of (1) **Cerebrum** (two cerebral hemispheres), the seat of the senses, mind and memory, and voluntary movement; (2) Hind brain comprising: the **cerebellum** or the little brain, concerned with balance, tone and muscular co-ordination, the **pons** or bridge and **medulla oblongata** or bulb, a prolongation of the spinal cord. The pons and medulla give origin to **12** pairs of **cranial nerves**.

The average **weight** of the human brain is 1.4 kgm (3 lbs) in an adult male and 0.1 kgm (¼ lb) less in an adult female.

The Spinal Cord

The spinal cord continues with the medulla downwards inside the vertebral canal. It is a bundle of nerve cells and fibres (neurons), issuing **31** pairs of nerves passing through spaces between the vertebrae to form spinal nerves, connective-tissue covered like pieces of white string. They are distributed to the internal organs, trunk and limbs.

All cranial and spinal nerves carry messages **to** the brain (**sensory** nerves) from the sense organs and the skin; and **from** the brain to the muscles, causing their motion (**motor** nerves). Restoration of a severed nerve takes some months to join.

The Autonomic Nervous System: two subdivisions

The larger subdivision, termed the Sympathetic system, whose chains, ganglia (collections of nerve cells) and the plexus (networks of nerve fibres) originate inside the chest and abdomen. The lesser subdivision, termed the Parasympathetic system, whose nerve cells arise from the hind brain (cerebellum, pons and medulla), join the cranial and spinal nerves with their fibres. There is also a visceral component.

The Autonomic Nervous System (Greek autos = self, nomos = law) spontaneously controls unstriped muscle tissue and is distributed in the various viscera: the heart, blood vessels, bowel, glands, urinary and reproductive organs.

44

The larger component of the Autonomic Nervous System: the Sympathetic

It originates from aggregate of nerve cells (ganglia, plural of ganglion). The cells' outgrowths form two chain-like nerve cords, lying on each side and in front of the vertebral column. They communicate with the spinal nerves of the Central Nervous System. They then proceed to form networks, the plexuses, of slender sympathetic nerves along the course of the large blood vessels and around the thoracic and abdominal viscera. The central part of each suprarenal gland, situated at top of each kidney and which secretes **adrenalin**, is made up of sympathetic nerve tissue and is under the control of that system.

Structural unit of the Nervous System

The structural unit or unit-cell, the single undivided entity, of the nervous system is the **nerve cell** or **neuron** with its protoplasmic outgrowths (fig. 13). These outgrowths are (a) **dendrites** (Greek = branches of tree), which are arborisation or processes forming connection with other nerve cells' outgrowths; (b) **axon** (Greek = axis), a long thread-like protoplasmic growth, bundles of which form a peripheral nerve (periphery = outer boundary).

Summary

The **Nervous System** is the principal regulator and director of all other systems. It receives communications (messages) from within, the internal environment, and from without, the external environment of the outside world. It responds either automatically or by design.

The next two systems to be dealt with in connection with physical exercise are the Cardiovascular System and Respiratory System. These will be preceded by a system of identifying the voluntary muscles of the body and their actions.

Chapter 8

SKELETAL MUSCLES —
THE BARE ESSENTIALS

For the purpose of simplicity and ease of remembering, (a) only the chief muscles are stated with their approximate attachments and (b) 'from' denotes the muscle origin and 'to' expresses its insertion, which is the place of attachment to the bone that the muscle moves. These will be followed by the muscle action, but no muscle acts in isolation.

Head

Two groups:
Muscles of expression, attached to skin.
Muscles of mastication.

Neck

Streno-mastoid: **from** sternum (breast bone), slanting up **to** mastoid bone, behind ear.
Action: draws head towards shoulder (fig. 19)

Trapezius: two flat triangular muscles, together form a trapezium, a quadrilateral figure with no two sides parallel (fig. 20), **from** occiput (back of skull) and vertebral spines of neck and thorax **to** back of clavicle (collar bone) and scapula (shoulder blade).

Action: draws head down to one side (fig. 19) or back (fig. 22); draws scapula up and down (fig. 21); when used as a whole, i.e., both sides, draws shoulders back (fig. 22).

In pursuance of the back, read on:

Latissimus dorsi (broadest of the back), fig. 20: **from** all lumbar and

47

SKELETAL MUSCLES

Bones are moved at joints by the CONTRACTION and RELAXATION of MUSCLES attached to them.

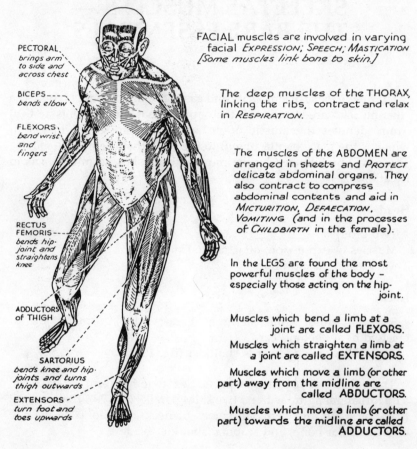

PECTORAL
brings arm to side and across chest

BICEPS
bends elbow

FLEXORS
bend wrist and fingers

RECTUS FEMORIS
bends hip-joint and straightens knee

ADDUCTORS of THIGH

SARTORIUS
bends knee and hip joints and turns thigh outwards

EXTENSORS
turn foot and toes upwards

FACIAL muscles are involved in varying facial *EXPRESSION; SPEECH; MASTICATION [Some muscles link bone to skin.]*

The deep muscles of the THORAX, linking the ribs, contract and relax in *RESPIRATION.*

The muscles of the ABDOMEN are arranged in sheets and *PROTECT* delicate abdominal organs. They also contract to compress abdominal contents and aid in *MICTURITION, DEFAECATION, VOMITING* (and in the processes of *CHILDBIRTH* in the female).

In the LEGS are found the most powerful muscles of the body – especially those acting on the hip-joint.

Muscles which bend a limb at a joint are called FLEXORS.

Muscles which straighten a limb at a joint are called EXTENSORS.

Muscles which move a limb (or other part) away from the midline are called ABDUCTORS.

Muscles which move a limb (or other part) towards the midline are called ADDUCTORS.

Figure 17

SKELETAL MUSCLES

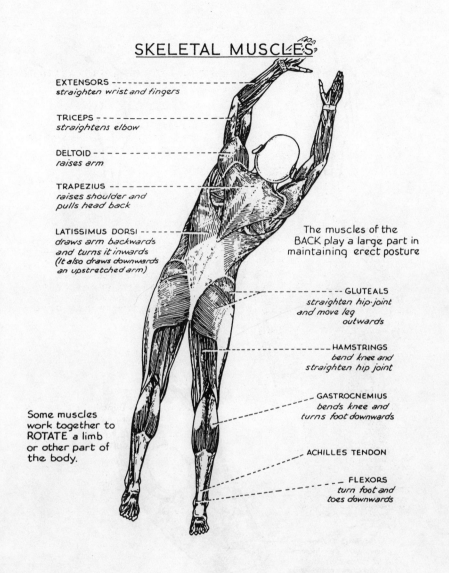

EXTENSORS -
straighten wrist and fingers

TRICEPS - - - - - - - - - - - - - - - - - -
straightens elbow

DELTOID - - - - - - - - - - - - - - - - -
raises arm

TRAPEZIUS - - - - - - - - - - - - - -
*raises shoulder and
pulls head back*

LATISSIMUS DORSI - - - - - - -
*draws arm backwards
and turns it inwards
(It also draws downwards
an upstretched arm)*

The muscles of the
BACK play a large part in
maintaining erect posture

- - - - - - GLUTEALS
*straighten hip-joint
and move leg
outwards*

- - - - HAMSTRINGS
*bend knee and
straighten hip joint*

GASTROCNEMIUS
*bends knee and
turns foot downwards*

Some muscles
work together to
ROTATE a limb
or other part of
the body.

ACHILLES TENDON

FLEXORS
*turn foot and
toes downwards*

Figure 18

49

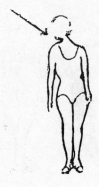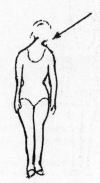

Figure 19

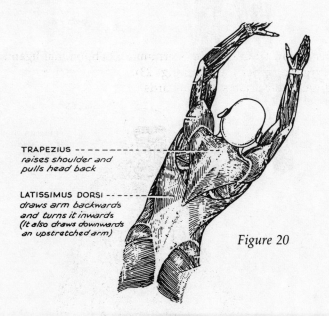

TRAPEZIUS - - - - - - - - - - - - - - - -
raises shoulder and
pulls head back

LATISSIMUS DORSI - - - - - - -
draws arm backwards
and turns it inwards
(It also draws downwards
an upstretched arm)

Figure 20

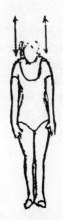 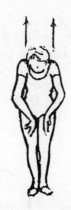 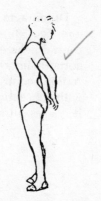

Figure 21   *Figure 22*

sacral vertebrae, and iliac crest, fibres converge out and up to inside upper humerus.

Action: adducts (draws towards the median axis of body) arm and draws it backwards (fig. 22).

Chest

Front

Pectoralis major: **from** clavicle, sternum and abdominal ligament, fibres converge to upper humerus (fig. 23).

Action: adducts and rotates arm inwards.

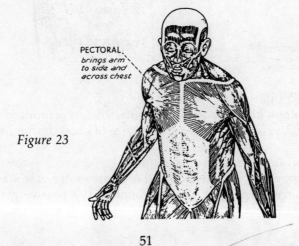

PECTORAL
brings arm
to side and
across chest

Figure 23

Muscles of respiration

Diaphragm: dome-shaped, dividing thorax from abdomen (fig. 24 and fig. 50); **from** sternum, lower ribs and lumbar vertebrae to a central ligament, with openings for passage of oesophagus (gullet), aorta (main artery of the body) and inferior vena cava (main vein). **Action**: contracts during inspiration and is flattened and lowered with consequent increase in the length (depth) of the thoracic cavity. It relaxes during expiration and assumes its dome shape.

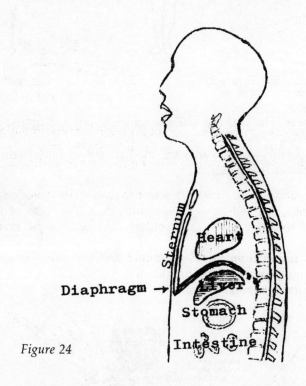

Figure 24

External intercostals (between ribs).
Action: draw ribs upwards and outwards, synchronous with the diaphragm's contraction, to increase size of chest during inspiration.

Internal intercostals (between ribs).
Action: draw ribs downwards and inwards to decrease size of chest during forced expiration. Quiet expiration is a passive gravitational movement.

Abdomen

Muscles of the abdominal wall

Rectus abdominis, in the middle of front of abdomen, **from** pubis to sternum (fig. 17), incorporating the umbilicus (navel) midway. **Action**: tightens abdomen (compresses it), also draws thorax down (figs. 25 and 26).

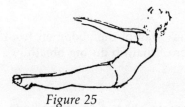

Figure 25

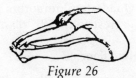

Figure 26

Obliquus externus abdominus and **obliquus internus abdominis**: the external forms the outer layer and the internal the inner. **Action**: both diminish capacity of abdomen (compress it), fig. 25.

Transversus abdominis: **from** iliac crest **to** inside the lower costal cartilages of ribs, lying deeply. Fibres run across the front of the abdomen and towards the back at either side behind the **rectus abdominis**. **Action**: bends thorax sideways (figs. 27 and 28).

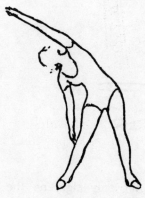

Figure 27

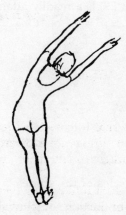

Figure 28

In the **groin**, the abdominal wall is traversed by the inguinal canal on either side, a common site for hernia (rupture), caused by sudden strain or rupture of muscles. Inguinal hernia occurs more in males than females. The inguinal canal permits the passage of a cord in either sex. In the male the cord suspends the testicle. In the female a cord passes from the uterus to the groin. The rupture may also exist from birth due to weakness of the abdominal wall as with an umbilical hernia. Part of an intestinal loop may be pushed into the inside opening of the inguinal canal, in the case of a rupture, causing acute intestinal obstruction.

Quadratus lumborum forms the back wall of the abdomen **from** iliac crest to twelfth rib and is a fixator of that rib during breathing.

Pelvic floor

From beneath the pubis and ischium on either side of the bone-fused pelvic girdle (fig. 1), muscle fibres are directed towards the midline. The large **levator ani** and the small **coccygeus** behind it are the two main muscles.

In the female, three openings are formed in the midline of the floor of the pelvis for the urethra, vagina and anus.

Astride horse-riding is one of the best exercises for strengthening the pelvic floor, since the levator ani muscle contracts in association with contraction of the adductors of the thighs. Scissor movement (fig. 29) is a readily attainable exemplification.

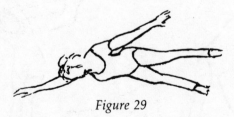

Figure 29

Muscles of the spine

Contraction of the abdominal muscles not only tightens the abdomen thereby compressing the viscera, but also flexes the trunk forward and sideways. It is the muscles of the back on either side of the vertebral column that support and extend this column and the back. Stretching exercises (figs. 30 to 35) are best for keeping the trunk erect and counterbalance the inescapable flexing and bending forward, the daily movements of the body are in the front.

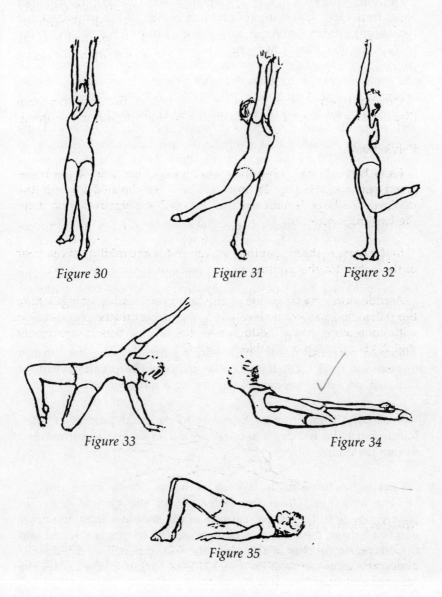

Figure 30

Figure 31

Figure 32

Figure 33

Figure 34

Figure 35

Muscles of the upper limb

Muscles of the upper arm include the **deltoid**, **biceps**, **brachialis** and **triceps** (figs. 17 and 18).

Deltoid: a thick triangular **V**-shaped muscle covering the shoulder joint, **from** clavicle and the rough outer border of the scapular spine (acromion), fibres converge to a rough knob-like area about the middle of outer side of humerus.
Action: it acts in part or as a whole, (a) the front part co-operates with the pectoralis major to draw the arm forward; (b) the back part co-operates with the latissimus dorsi to draw the arm outwards and backwards with the aid of the supraspinatus muscle underneath it, it abducts (pulls away from the body's midline) at right angle with the body, at the shoulder joint. To raise the arm up further requires the co-operation of the trapezius (fig. 18). Both the deltoid and trapezius move the clavicle and scapula slightly up towards the head as the arm is raised right up.

Biceps: has two heads of origin, the short head **from** outer process of scapula, the long head from above the glenoid cavity which receives the head of the humerus (figs. 8 and 5), in conjunction with the fibrous capsule of the shoulder joint but *within* that capsule. The fusiform-shaped body of the biceps muscle tapers to a flattened tendon, to be inserted into a rough area of the upper end of radius (the outer bone of the forearm) after crossing the elbow joint, opposite the bend of the elbow.
Action: a powerful flexor of the elbow joint, drawing the forearm towards the arm (fig. 8). It is also a supinator of the forearm twisting it outward, an action needed when turning a screw or nut.

Brachialis: **from** front of humerus to coranoid process of ulna. Jointly with the biceps, it is a prime mover of the forearm when flexing the elbow joint.

Triceps: has three heads. It occupies the back of the upper arm (fig. 8). The long head **from** the lower rim of the glenoid cavity in conjunction with the fibrous capsule of the shoulder joint; the other two heads **from** the back of the humerus. The triceps is inserted into the olecranon process of the ulna, the funny bone, so called since hitting the ulnar nerve at the inner side of back of elbow causes the "funny sensations".

Action: extends the elbow joint.

Muscles of forearm and hand

The front is occupied by the **flexors** of wrist and fingers, requiring no great effort. The back is occupied by the **extensors**. The short muscles of the hand include flexors of thumb, abductors and adductors of all five digits.

Many figures in this chapter and elsewhere illustrate almost all movements of the upper limbs.

Muscles of the lower limb

Muscles of lower limb are of course much larger and stronger than those of the upper limb.

Thigh

Front

Iliopsoas (iliacus and psoas): **from** iliac bones and vertebral column **to** the lesser trochater of femur, on each side.
Action: flexion and abduction of hip joints (figs. 36, 37, 38, 39 and 40).

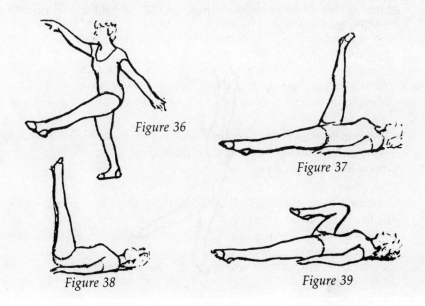

Figure 36

Figure 37

Figure 38

Figure 39

Adductors of thigh: these are three triangular muscles (fig. 17) placed in the groin below the iliopsoas, **from** pubis, fanning out **to** inner aspect of femur.

Action: adducts thigh at hip joint (fig. 40 shows adduction and flexion at hip joint).

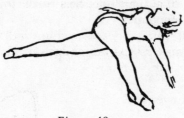

Figure 40

Sartorius, longest muscle in body (fig. 17), **from** front tip of iliac crest, crossing the front of thigh obliquely downwards to tibia.

Action: assists in flexing hip and knee joints and in rotating thigh inwards.

Quadriceps femoris (led by the rectus femoris, fig. 17): a fleshy mass of four muscles, mainly **from** shaft of femur **to** patella (knee cap).

Action: extend the knee joint (figs. 34, 37, 40 and 41), promoting standing and kicking!

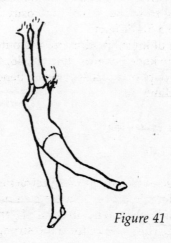

Figure 41

Back

Gluteals, a group of three muscles (fig. 18): gluteus maximus, medius and minimus, mainly **from** upper and outer dorsum (back surface) of ilium, sacrum and coccyx. Fibres run obliquely downwards and outwards **to** the greater trochanter of femur. The lower and deep fibres of **gluteus maximus** run **to** a rough area below the lesser trochater of femur.

Action: maximus extends thigh; medius abducts and rotates thigh outwards; minimus abducts thigh (figs. 41, 42, 43 and 44).

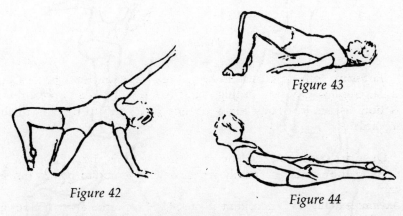

Figure 43

Figure 42

Figure 44

Hamstrings, so called because of their strong tendons or strings (fig. 18), easily felt on either side of the back of the knee (two inners and one outer), **from** the ischial tuberosity, what you sit on, **to** outer top ends of tibia and fibula.

Action: flexion of knee; in addition, the outer rotates knee outwards; the inners rotate knee inwards (figs. 45, 46, 47 and 48). The three form a powerful group of muscles which bends the knee in walking, jumping and climbing.

Muscles of the lower leg

Muscles of the calf

The two muscles of the calf, the **gastrocnemius** (fig. 18) and **soleus**, possess considerable power. **Gastrocnemius from** condyles of femur at either side of knee, **soleus**, in front of gastrocnemius, **from** back of tibia and fibula. They join to form the strong **tendo Achilles** (Achilles was a Greek warrior whose vulnerability was the heel). The Achilles tendon is inserted into the back of the heel bone (fig. 18).

Action: the gastrocnemius is the propelling force in walking, running and leaping. The soleus is the steadying force of the leg in the standing position, particularly if on one leg.

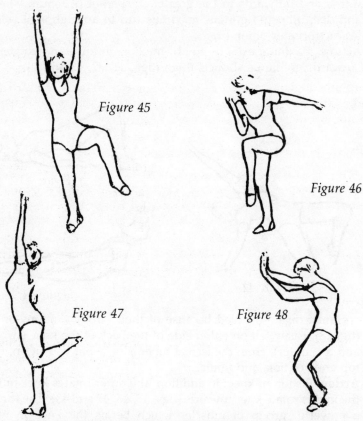

Figure 45

Figure 46

Figure 47

Figure 48

When the heel is raised by the contraction of the two muscles, it moves away from the ball of the foot and a hardly noticeable extension or straightening takes place. This is restricted by the strong **plantar aponeurosis** (plantar = relating to the sole of the foot), which is a robust fibrous sheet, playing a subsidiary part in maintaining the longitudinal (front to back) arches of the foot. It is the short muscles of the sole, i.e., plantar aspect, which play the major part in maintaining both the transverse and the longitudinal arches. If this aponeurosis and the other ligaments which protect the arches become weakened or overstretched, from any cause, then the bones which form the arches sink down, and a flat foot results.

Tibialis anterior: from outer side of tibia, the upper half is fleshy, the lower tendinous. The long tendon makes its way towards the inner side of the foot **to** the internal cuneiform bone and the base of first metatarsal.
Action: it everts the foot, turning the inner side outwards. It also assists in maintaining balance when standing.

Extensors of the toes have similar construction as those of the fingers. They are inserted into the phalanges. They extend the toes, i.e., raise them up.

Inference: any useful muscular exercise should include the renewed contraction of all the above muscles.

Summary

The two main movers of the head and shoulder blades are the sternomastoid and trapezius.

The diaphragm and intercostals are the muscles of respiration. Abdominal muscles bend thorax forward and sideways. They tighten the abdomen, *strengthening its wall*, and assist bowel movement.

The deltoid and trapezius raise the arm at the shoulder joint. The biceps and brachialis flex and triceps extends the elbow joint. Their exercise is beneficial and serviceable in daily life.

Muscles of the front of the thigh include the iliopsoas which flexes the hip and the quadriceps femoris which extends the knee. The sartorius rotates thigh outwards and assists in flexing the hip; the adductors move the thigh towards the midline.

The gluteals extend, abduct and rotate the thigh. The hamstrings flex and rotate the knee. The powerful muscles of the calf are the propelling force in walking, running and leaping.

This chapter has dealt with the bare essentials of the **skeletal musculature** *including muscles of respiration which play a major part in the state of our oxygenation and fitness. The next chapter will deal with the* **mechanics of respiration**, *which follows in due order. This will show that expansion of the thorax by the contraction of the diaphragm and external intercostals, creates a vacuum where a space containing gas below atmospheric pressure, leads to* *suction of air into the lungs. The lungs play a passive mechanical role with the abdominal wall acting as a co-ordinator, and quiet expiration (not forced) is a tranquil gravitational action.*

Exercises

What immediately follows is (a) a memory exercise, and (b) a suggested daily ten-minute physical exercise.

(a) Memory exercise

Name the main muscles acting in the following 46 illustrated movements. Scoring 25, which is more than 50%, is considered good, above 30 is very good and above 40 is excellent.

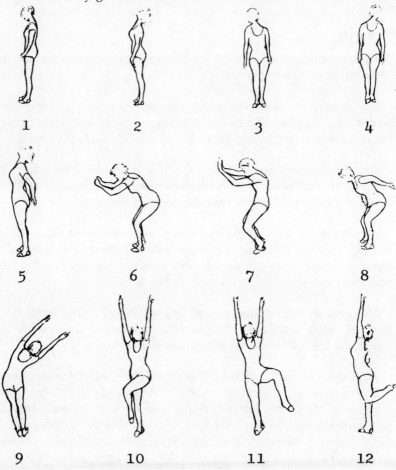

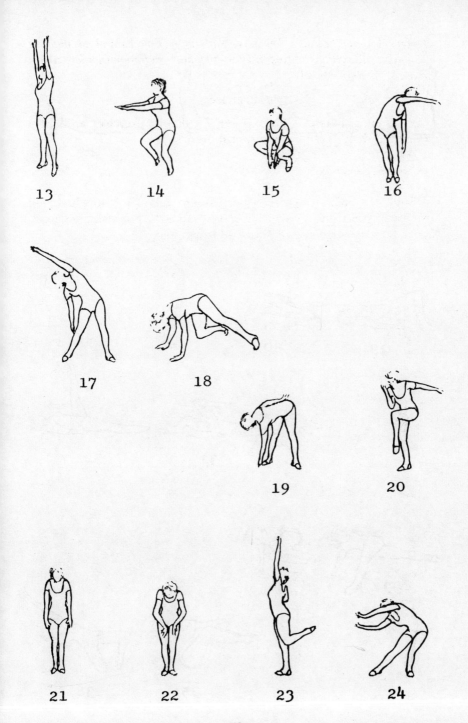

13   14   15   16

17   18

19   20

21   22   23   24

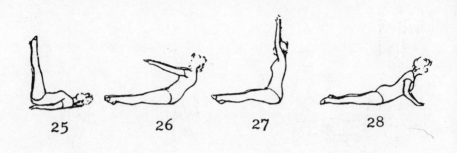

25   26   27   28

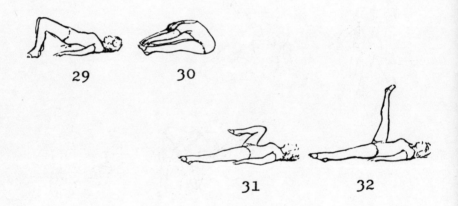

29   30

31   32

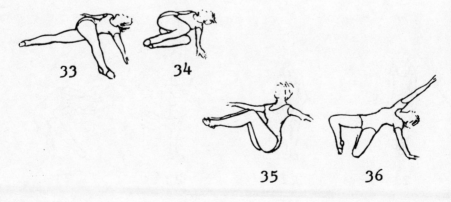

33   34

35   36

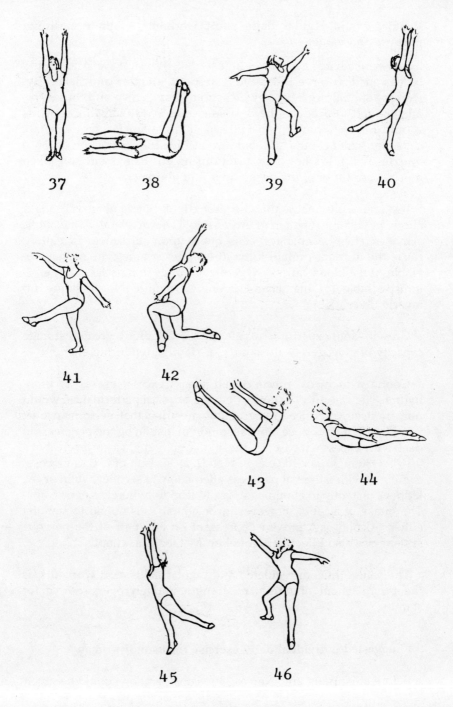

37   38   39   40

41   42

43   44

45   46

Regulated and regular daily short workouts — their meaning, purpose and value

To be effective as a means of fitness, daily physical exercises should be designed to serve three ends: **strength, stamina** and **flexibility**. Exercise should not be so severe as to defeat its own end, but vigorous enough to produce the desired result. Worthwhile movements should not only have strong internal muscle tension by deliberate active muscular contraction, but also include the contraction of those muscles which are not often used during our daily avocation. Such muscles are those of the **back, sides** and **abdomen**.

It is relevant to realise that the **strength** of muscle fibres is brought about by their growth and expansion. The accelerated metabolic activities (chemical changes) consequent upon quickened circulation, cause the nutrient **protein** to build up muscle fibre. The oxyhaemoglobin of the blood carries oxygen from lungs to muscles. Oxygen is indispensable for that chemical energy required for building up muscle fibres.

Growth and expansion of muscle fibres afford greater storage capacity of **glycogen** — the source of **stamina** (enduring energy).

Contrary to many preconceived ideas, excess intake of carbohydrate such as glucose shortly before a physical performance, would not, by itself, produce greater stamina during that performance. It would certainly produce more secretion of insulin by the pancreas, to deal with excess glucose in the blood. Blood-glucose level above 0.18% (180 mgm per 100 c.c. of blood), as a result of excess glucose, combined with failure of pancreas adequately to secrete insulin or the kidneys instantly to eliminate it, could lead to hyperglycaemic coma. The intake of alcohol, however inconsiderable, is no aid to stamina either. Alcohol is a proven depressant on any part of the nervous system (see also Effect of Alcohol on Metabolism, chapter 12).

The value, thus, of regulated and regular daily short workouts, is the improvement of muscular strength and glycogen reserve for stamina.

(b) **Suggested individual daily exercise for man or woman**

Before attempting any exercise, due consideration should be given to (1) **timing**, (2) **duration**, (3) **successive stages**, which take into account (a) your present limitations and age, (b) number of movement repetitions, (c) exercising both sides of the body, where applicable, (d) to discontinue at any feeling of 'stress' or shortness of breath, and (e) the procedure.

Timing

Early morning or late evening, before a meal, not immediately afterwards, maybe followed by a bath or shower.

Duration

5 minutes daily for the first week, 10 for the second and 15 or more for the third and subsequent weeks.

Successive stages

'Warming up' for 1–2 minutes, to increase blood supply to muscles, prior to intensified activity and internal muscle tension. 'Warming up' can be effected by walking round the room; flexing or stretching or swinging arms and legs; jogging in place; walking up or downstairs and back.

'Warming up' is followed by a ready workout programme. Two programmes are offered, (1) a starting and (2) more advanced one. Variations can be made from the illustrated movements in the present chapter, as you progress.

Each movement should be repeated 8 times (to include each side, where applicable). The number of repetitions should be increased as fitness develops.

SUGGESTED STARTING PROGRAMME

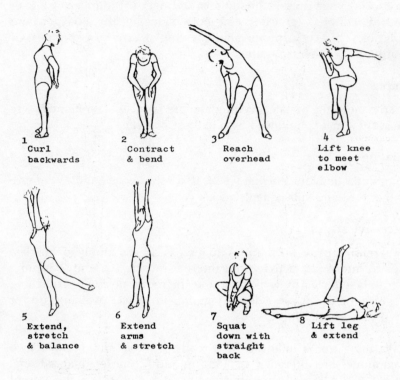

1 Curl backwards

2 Contract & bend

3 Reach overhead

4 Lift knee to meet elbow

5 Extend, stretch & balance

6 Extend arms & stretch

7 Squat down with straight back

8 Lift leg & extend

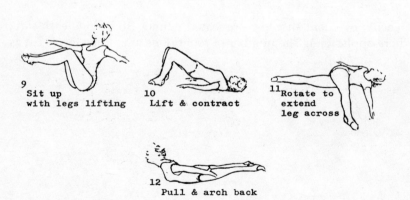

9 Sit up with legs lifting

10 Lift & contract

11 Rotate to extend leg across

12 Pull & arch back

A MORE ADVANCED PROGRAMME

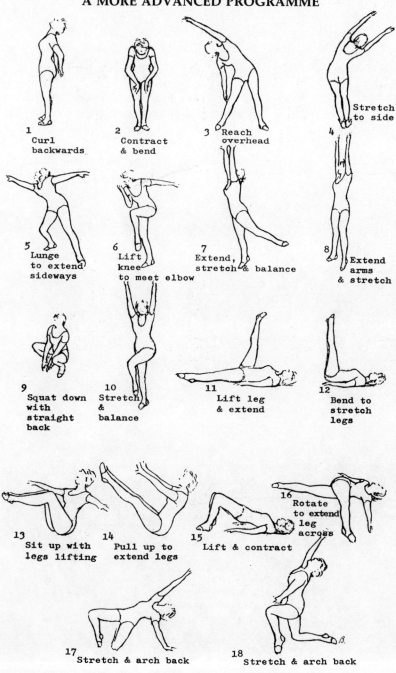

1 Curl backwards

2 Contract & bend

3 Reach overhead

4 Stretch to side

5 Lunge to extend sideways

6 Lift knee to meet elbow

7 Extend, stretch & balance

8 Extend arms & stretch

9 Squat down with straight back

10 Stretch & balance

11 Lift leg & extend

12 Bend to stretch legs

13 Sit up with legs lifting

14 Pull up to extend legs

15 Lift & contract

16 Rotate to extend leg across

17 Stretch & arch back

18 Stretch & arch back

69

Chapter 9

RESPIRATION —
THE ACT OF BREATHING

Would you like to know what this show is all about before it is out? Have you ever wondered what is this breathing mass, named corpus? What is this living matter?

What is protoplasm?

Protoplasm (Greek protos = first, plasma = tangible thing formed) is the material basis of life in animals and plants. It is the physical part of man as distinct from mind and spirit. It is the sustenance of every living cell (fig. 13).

Protoplasm has been known for almost a century to contain the elements of carbon, nitrogen, oxygen, hydrogen. It is composed also of other varied complex compounds, depending on the type of tissue, containing the elements of **iron, phosphorus, sulphur, calcium, potassium, sodium, chlorine and magnesium**.

Oxygen — a reactive gaseous element

Oxygen is not only a constituent element of protoplasm, but the very instrument of its formation. It readily reacts, oxidises, combusts or combines with all these elements. In fact 50% of the earth's crust is composed of oxygen. 21% of the atmospheric air we breathe is composed of oxygen, becoming 14% of the alveolar air in contact with the respiratory epithelium, in the depths of the lungs, which carries out gaseous exchanges with the blood.

Inspired air is composed of 21% O_2, 79% N, 0.04% CO_2
Expired air is composed of 16.5% O_2, 79.5% N, 4% CO_2
Alveolar air is composed of 14% O_2, 80.5% N, 5.5% CO_2

The **tidal air** flowing in and ebbing out like the tide, i.e., entering

71

and leaving the lungs with each cycle of respiration, every 3 seconds, is about 400 c.c., and the **dead space air**, occupying the conducting air passages of larynx, trachea, main bronchi and bronchioles, is about 140 c.c. Respiratory **rate** is about 18 cycles per minute.

Oxygen, thus, is essential to life, a nutriment absorbed into the blood (haemoglobin becomes oxyhaemoglobin), transported to the tissues to construct molecules for energy **storage** or **release**, for **growth** or **movement**.

The two manifestations of life

Growth and movement are the two manifestations of life, without which life lessens and wastes. When oxygen is used up by the cells, CO_2 is given off as a toxic waste-product, carried by the blood **plasma** to the lungs and is disposed of in the expired air.

Respiration

Respiration is the natural action of breathing. The process of exchanging gases **twice**: in the lungs, termed **external respiration**; in the tissues, where oxygen is actually used up, termed **internal respiration**.

External or lung respiration(fig. 49)

External respiration is the process of taking up oxygen by the pulmonary veins (4 veins, 2 to each lung, fig. 52) from the inspired air (alveolar oxygen is about 14% of alveolar air). The **oxygenated** blood is carried to the **left** auricle of the heart, pumped out by the **left** ventricle into the aorta and distributed to the tissues.

The **de-oxygenated** blood, carrying CO_2 in the plasma, mainly in the form of bicarbonate, from the tissues to the **right** auricle, is pumped out by the **right** ventricle into the pulmonary arteries (1 for each lung) to the lungs. The CO_2 is then released in the expired air.

It will not have escaped you that the pulmonary veins are the only veins in the body which return **oxygenated** blood to the heart and the pulmonary arteries are the only arteries which carry **de**-oxygenated blood from the heart.

The act of association and dissociation of oxygen, which is carried

RESPIRATORY SYSTEM

All living cells require to get OXYGEN from the fluid around them and to get rid of CARBON DIOXIDE to it.

INTERNAL RESPIRATION is the exchange of these gases between tissue cells and their fluid environment.

EXTERNAL RESPIRATION is the exchange of these gases *(oxygen and carbon dioxide)* between the body and the external environment.

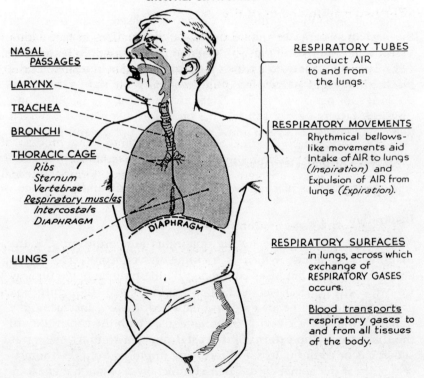

NASAL PASSAGES

LARYNX

TRACHEA

BRONCHI

THORACIC CAGE
 Ribs
 Sternum
 Vertebrae
 Respiratory muscles
 Intercostals
 DIAPHRAGM

LUNGS

DIAPHRAGM

RESPIRATORY TUBES
 conduct AIR
 to and from
 the lungs.

RESPIRATORY MOVEMENTS
 Rhythmical bellows-like movements aid
 Intake of AIR to lungs
 (Inspiration) and
 Expulsion of AIR from
 lungs *(Expiration)*.

RESPIRATORY SURFACES
 in lungs, across which
 exchange of
 RESPIRATORY GASES
 occurs.

Blood transports
 respiratory gases to
 and from all tissues
 of the body.

Figure 49

out by the haemoglobin, the uptake and release of CO_2 by the plasma and the transfer of both O_2 and CO_2 is controlled chemically and nervously. The most important factor is the level of CO_2 in the blood passing through the **respiratory centres** in the hind brain (pons and medulla oblongata), which leads to alteration in the outgoing impulses to the respiratory **muscles**: the **diaphragm** and **intercostals** (fig. 50). There are, of course, voluntary and involuntary alterations in breathing, e.g., psychic or emotional influences.

Internal or tissue respiration

Internal respiration, where the oxygen is utilised, is the process of the exchange of gases between the capillaries (the minute blood vessels) and the tissues (fig. 53). Oxygen passes from blood to tissue cells. The CO_2 produced by the oxidation of carbon is carried by the blood to the **right** auricle. It is pumped out by the **right** ventricle to the lungs for removal (fig. 52). There are chemical, e.g., acidity, and physical factors, e.g., saturation, pressure, temperature, which determine levels of oxygen and CO_2 and their uptake and release.

Mechanics of the external respiration

Respiration takes place in two stages: **inspiration** and **expiration**.

Inspiration

With the 12th rib fixed by the quadratus lumborum muscle, the **diaphragm**, a dome, which is a prime mover, contracts. This is effected by motor impulses conducted by the phrenic nerve (mainly from the 4th cervical segment of the spinal cord). Its contraction causes the dome to be lowered and flattened, thereby increasing the **height** of the thoracic cavity. Simultaneously with the contraction of the diaphragm, the **external intercostal** muscles contract, acting as synergists or co-ordinators and receiving impulses from the thoracic segments of the spinal cord. Their contraction **expands** the chest by drawing the ribs upwards and outwards. The lungs expand to fill the space created by the diaphragm and intercostals and air is drawn in.

The abdominal wall moves **out** with inspiration.

Expiration

This is a passive action, helped by the gravitational force during quiet breathing. The diaphragm merely relaxes and assumes its

THORAX

The Thorax (*or* chest) is the closed cavity which contains the LUNGS, HEART and Great Vessels.

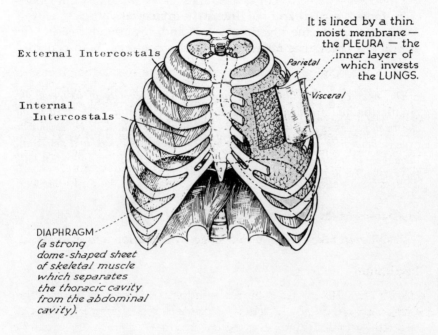

It is lined by a thin moist membrane — the PLEURA — the inner layer of which invests the LUNGS.

External Intercostals

Parietal

Visceral

Internal Intercostals

DIAPHRAGM
(a strong dome-shaped sheet of skeletal muscle which separates the thoracic cavity from the abdominal cavity).

DIMENSIONS of thoracic cage and the PRESSURE between pleural surfaces change rhythmically about 18-20 times a minute with the MOVEMENTS of RESPIRATION —— AIR MOVEMENT in and out of the lungs follows
                                                                                    passively.

Figure 50

75

original lax dome-like shape. At the same time the external inter-costals relax and ribs are lowered. Recoiling and shrinking of lungs expel the CO_2-laden air, conducted through the bronchi, trachea, larynx, pharynx, nose or mouth.

The abdominal wall moves **in** with expiration.

In **forced expiration**, the **internal intercostal** muscles actively contract, drawing the ribs downwards and inwards, decreasing the size of the chest. The abdominal muscles compress both abdomen and chest.

The next chapter will attempt to show how the state of oxygenation, **circulation** *and drainage of waste-products can determine the speed of the chemical processes in the body — metabolism. It will also endeavour to explain how prior physical exercises lead to* **energy storage** *and determine the degree of future* **strength** *and* **stamina** *or fitness. It will also deal with the mechanics of the* **cardiac pump**.

Chapter 10

THE CARDIOVASCULAR SYSTEM — HEART AND BLOOD CIRCULATION

This chapter begins the consideration of the one system upon which all other systems depend for their performance, indeed for their very existence, and is the source of life (fig. 51).

Movement begins with the pacemaker of the heart. Oxygen and nutriments are moved round the body by the cardiovascular system.

The heart

The heart is the rhythmic muscular **pump** with an automatic action which drives blood in circulation round the body.

It is the non-stop working which renders the heart the most important single organ in the body. Inherent impulses are discharged rhythmically from the **pacemaker**, a node of differentiated tissue in the right auricle (atrium). In fact, we are adhering to life now with our last muscle — the heart.

Your heart

In order that you may keep constantly before you a clear picture of the heart and what is set out below, it will be useful to think of your **own** left and right sides. The illustration depicts the heart of a person facing you (see diagram, fig. 52).

A non-communicating septum

The heart is divided into **two halves**, left and right, by a non-communicating septum (partition). There are two chambers to each half of the heart, making **four** in all. Above is a thin-walled auricle to

CARDIOVASCULAR SYSTEM

The CIRCULATORY System.   Chief TRANSPORT System
                                           of the body

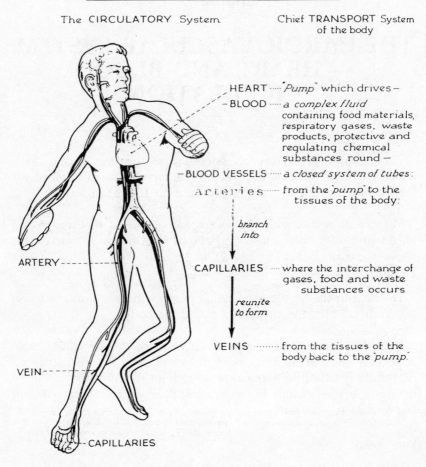

HEART ···· *"Pump"* which drives —

— BLOOD ···· a *complex fluid*
containing food materials,
respiratory gases, waste
products, protective and
regulating chemical
substances round —

— BLOOD VESSELS ···· a *closed system of tubes*:

Arteries ···· from the *"pump"* to the
tissues of the body:

*branch
into*

CAPILLARIES ···· where the interchange of
gases, food and waste
substances occurs

*reunite
to form*

VEINS ········ from the tissues of the
body back to the *"pump".*

ARTERY ------

VEIN ----

--CAPILLARIES

Figure 51

HEART

This is a *diagrammatic* section through the heart.

<u>HEART VALVES</u> have a core of Fibrous Tissue- - - - - - - - - -
covered on both sides with *Endothelium*

Extensions from
<u>AURICULO-VENTRICULAR (A-V)</u>
<u>FIBROUS RING</u>

Designed to
allow blood
to flow in
one direction
only —
from AURICLE
to VENTRICLE—
and on into
ARTERIES

The A-V valves
are attached by
thin CHORDAE
  TENDINEAE
    to
extensions of
CARDIAC MUSCLE—
PAPILLARY MUSCLES

These contract
when ventricles contract
and pull on Chordae
Tendineae so that valve
flaps cannot be everted.

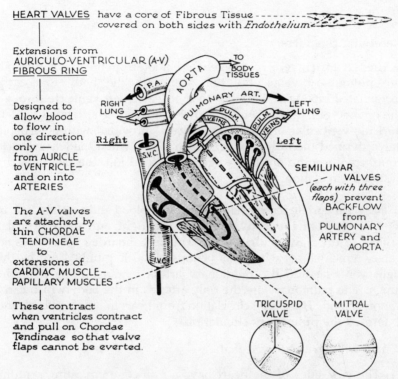

TO
BODY
TISSUES

AORTA

P.A.

PULMONARY ART.

RIGHT
LUNG

LEFT
LUNG

PULM.
VEINS

PULM.
VEINS

Right

Left

S.V.C.

I.V.C.

SEMILUNAR
VALVES
*(each with three
flaps)* prevent
BACKFLOW
from
PULMONARY
ARTERY and
AORTA.

TRICUSPID
VALVE

MITRAL
VALVE

*The Great Veins do not have valves guarding their entrance to the heart.
Thickening and contraction of the muscle around their mouths
prevent BACKFLOW of blood from heart.*

Figure 52

each side, and below are the thicker-walled ejecting **muscular ventricles**.

The **left** ventricle pumps out **oxygenated** blood into the **aorta**, the main artery of the body, and the **right** ventricle pumps out **de**-oxygenated blood into the arteries of the lung, the pulmonary arteries.

Receiving chambers

The **left auricle** receives oxygenated blood from the lungs, through the pulmonary veins, the only veins in the body that carry oxygenated blood, delivering it to the dilated **left ventricle** through the opened orifice between the auricle and ventricle, termed the left auriculo-venticular orifice. This orifice is provided with a **bi**cuspid valve, termed the **mitral** valve, which closes when the left ventricle contracts, to pump out the oxygenated blood into the aorta, for the **systemic** circulation.

The **right auricle** receives **de**-oxygenated blood and carrying CO_2 in its plasma from the body, through the right auriculo-ventricular orifice, to the **right ventricle**. This orifice is guarded by a **tri**cuspid valve, which closes when this venous blood is pumped out by the right ventricle into the pulmonary arteries, transporting it to the lungs. The pulmonary are the only arteries in the body which carry venous blood. This blood circulation from heart to lung and back and is termed the **pulmonary circulation**.

You will have observed that

(1) The two sides of the heart have a non-communicating septum, making the heart a concurrently-acting **double pump**.
(2) The left-side carries oxygenated blood and the right-side de-oxygenated venous blood.
(3) The two auricles receive their respective blood simultaneously and pass their respective blood to their ventricles at the same time. The two ventricles, of **equal capacity**, contract synchronously as if one entity, pumping their respective blood concurrently. The heart is, in fact, a double pump.

Main features of the heart

1. It has a pear-**shaped** appearance with narrow end below, termed the apex (fig. 52).

2. Base to apex **measures** about 12 cm (5 inches).

3. It **weighs** about 142 gm (9 ounces).

4. It **lies** at an angle, in a sloping position, with the apex pointing towards the **L.** hip and the base (broad end) facing the **R.** shoulder.

5. ⅔rds of the heart lies to the left of the **middle line** and ⅓rd to the right of it.

6. The heart is in a well-protected **position** in the thorax, and covered by a firm fibro-serous membrane, the **pericardium**, which is a two-layered closed sac, inside which is a moistening fluid.

7. The pericardium restrains the **overdistension** of the heart and is itself securely anchored to the diaphragm, back of breast bone and the roots of the great vessels.

8. The heart **beats** about 72 beats per minute, at rest. The period of contraction is termed **systole**, that of dilatation, **diastole**. The complete cycle lasts about 0.8 second (divide 60 into 72). Heart beat constitutes the **pulse**, best felt at the wrist, just above the root of the thumb, where the end of the radial artery lies near the surface on the radial bone.

9. With the heart at rest, beating 72 per minute, 5 litres of **blood** are delivered by each ventricle per minute. **250 c.c.** of **oxygen** are delivered by the **left ventricle** each minute or **70 cc.** per beat (5000/72).

10. The heart beat is best **heard** in the 5th intercostal space to the left of the sternum, the breast bone.

11. The **pacemaker** initiates and maintains the normal heart beat. The **heart rate** is altered by many influences: exercise, emotion, adrenalin, drugs, etc. There is a **nervous** regulation as well. Impulses are discharged to the heart from the **autonomic** nervous system: from (a) the medulla oblongata, in the hind brain, through the vagus nerve and (b) the thoracic sympathetic chain.

Effect of exercise on the heart

A more **powerful heart beat** results from regular and regulated exercise, most likely due to better coronary circulation (circulation in the heart muscles themselves). A competent muscular heart improves the whole circulation of the body (fig. 53), not only of blood, but lymph, which accelerates tissue circulation and with it the chemical changes (metabolism). Lymph removes any excess fluid of protein, thereby permitting fresh fluid from the blood. The lymphatic system is also a source of supply of lymphocytes (white blood cells) and lymph glands entrap harmful bacteria. Red and other white cells are formed by the bone marrow.

GENERAL COURSE of the CIRCULATION

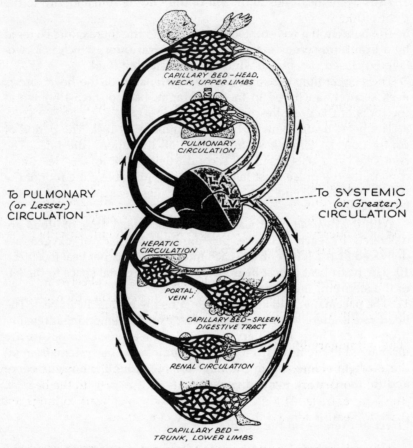

Figure 53

It is well to emphasise that the increased oxygen-carrying power of blood is the result, not only of a healthy vigorous heart, but also of expanded oxygen intake by the lungs.

Development of muscles from improved circulation serves to enlarge them. Trained enlarged muscles possess more protein and glycogen than the untrained, which afford expansion of their muscle-fibres with protein and greater storage capacity of glycogen.

The systemic blood circulation

Contraction of the left ventricle propels blood to all parts of the body through a widely-spread series of tubes, termed **arteries**. These branch into smaller ones, termed **arterioles**, then into tiny **capillaries** of microscopic dimension. These supply the tissues with oxygen and nutriments. Chemical changes take place in the cells of the tissues, termed **metabolism** (Greek metabole = change). These changes are either converting substances into living form: anabolism (Greek ana = up) **or** breaking down intricate matter into simpler substances to produce energy: catabolism (Greek Kata = down). In either case waste products are usually produced such as CO_2.

CO_2 is carried by the blood plasma. Blood is collected into tiny vessels, termed **venules** which unite to form **veins**, then to larger veins, which return the blood to the **right ventricle**.

The pulmonary blood circulation

The **right ventricle** pumps out venous blood to the lungs, through the pulmonary arteries. After oxygenation, it returns to the heart, to the left ventricle. The movement of blood from heart to lungs and back to heart is termed the pulmonary circulation.

Fitness is largely dependent on a powerful heart, accelerated oxygenation and tissue circulation. This cannot be achieved without the body's musculature: heart muscle, blood vessels, viscera and skeletal muscles. Muscles in turn are dependent for their health on effective nutritition, which means **a well-balanced diet**. *This will be the subject of the proceeding chapters.*

Chapter 11

EFFECTIVE NUTRITION

Nutrition is the foremost function of living plants and animals, consisting of the constant taking in of food and its subsequent assimilation into the body.

Regularity and regulation are natural activities occurring normally inside living organisms through chemical changes of substances taken in, whereby tissues are uniformally formed and energy is liberated.

In the human body the successive highly organised, methodically arranged stages are termed mastication, deglutition, digestion, absorption, assimilation and excretion. Excretion is produced by expiration, perspiration, urination and defecation. Nature and health: conditions of body and mind in which all the functions are regularly performed, demand orderly and controlled nutrition which is the subject that comes next.

A WELL BALANCED DIET

No love is more sincere than the love of food — to eat is human, to be healthy, divine. To make the most of it you will need to regulate your food and that is **diet**.

The principal aim of this exposition is to promote and sustain good health. An adequate understanding of what happens to food when absorbed should be clear before venturing on a course of a healthy diet.

Metabolism

Nutrition is the main source of metabolism. Without a mother's constructive metabolism, arising from nourishment, there would be no new life. The young body of the unborn is the product of an internal biochemical creation — metabolism.

Metabolism is the continual **chemical change** in the living body which takes place during circulation, respiration, digestion, secretion, movement, growth, repair and regeneration.

It comprises: (a) **constructive** metabolism: the process of converting nutritive substances into living form; (b) **destructive** metabolism: the process of breaking down intricate living matter into spent simpler substances.

What influences these chemical processes in the living body?

In addition to **nutrition**, other factors affect metabolism: age, body-surface area, atmospheric and body temperature, drugs and disease, but more significantly: (1) the body ductless **glands**, largely the thyroid, adrenal and pituitary, and above all (2) muscular work (**movement**).

Nutriments and muscular exercise

Trained muscles store in their cells more energy-producing **carbo-hydrate** (glycogen) than the untrained, generating **stamina** (power of endurance) and vitality. Vitamins also provide stamina through resisting infection and deficiency disorders.

Whereas carbohydrate and vitamins are necessary for endurance, **protein** is indispensible for **strength**. The main function of protein, however, is not an energy source, but cell-building and replacement.

Fat is an energy **reserve**. If there is no exertion, fat acts as an added padding agent. "Fatties" it is true, amply match a description sometimes used: "She looked as if she had been poured into her clothes and had forgotten to say when". The stored fat referred to here is the conspicuous subcutaneous adipose tissue, whose source is mainly the fat in the food.

During exercise, muscle glycogen (muscle mainly is made up of protein) breaks down into lactic acid which is neutralised into lactate by the alkaline blood-plasma, to be combusted by oxygen to yield $CO_2 + H_2O$ + heat + energy. This chemical energy is converted into mechanical energy, not unlike the combustion of fuel-oil to produce mechanical power. Metabolism, as well as oxygen consumption, may multiply 10 times or more during muscular exercise.

The role of ductless glands

Secretion of ductless glands varies with each individual. We are not made alike. **Thyroxin**, the active iodine compound, is secreted by the thyroid gland, which is situated on each side of the front of the neck. **Adrenalin**, which converts glycogen stored in liver into glucose, is secreted by the adrenal glands (suprarenals), situated at the top of each kidney. These two secretions, thyroxin and adrenalin, **directly** accelerate metabolism.

The **pituitary** is the leader of the endocrine orchestra (thyroid, parathyroid, adrenal and thymus) see fig. 54. These ductless glands: also termed endrocine glands, produce **hormones**, which pass directly from their cells into the blood stream. Hormones are chemical substances, each is formed in one organ, carried by the blood stream to another part which it stimulates. There are other hormone-producing cells inside certain organs — ovary, testis; pancreas (producing insulin).

The pituitary gland, situated at the base of the brain, performs **indirectly**. Its thyrotropic hormone indirectly raises metabolism by acting on the thyroid gland.

The special role of the adrenal gland

The adrenal gland plays an important role during our physical and mental activities.

Each adrenal gland is made up of two parts: an outer **cortex** and a central **medulla**:

(1) The active hormone of the gland's cortex, **cortin**, is essential to life and has a great capacity for absorbing vitamin C. The adrenotropic hormone of the **pituitary** controls the activity of the adrenal cortex.
(2) The active hormone of the gland's medulla is **adrenalin**. The adrenal medulla is developed from, connected to and influenced by, the sympathetic nervous system, and under adverse emotional stress is stimulated by that system.

ENDOCRINE SYSTEM

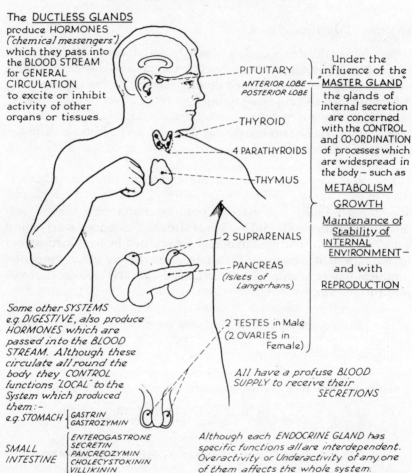

The <u>DUCTLESS GLANDS</u> produce HORMONES ("chemical messengers") which they pass into the BLOOD STREAM for GENERAL CIRCULATION to excite or inhibit activity of other organs or tissues.

PITUITARY
ANTERIOR LOBE
POSTERIOR LOBE

THYROID

4 PARATHYROIDS

THYMUS

2 SUPRARENALS

PANCREAS
(Islets of Langerhans)

2 TESTES in Male
(2 OVARIES in Female)

Under the influence of the "MASTER GLAND" the glands of internal secretion are concerned with the CONTROL and CO-ORDINATION of processes which are widespread in the body – such as

METABOLISM

GROWTH

Maintenance of Stability of INTERNAL ENVIRONMENT –

and with

REPRODUCTION.

All have a profuse BLOOD SUPPLY to receive their SECRETIONS

Some other SYSTEMS e.g. DIGESTIVE, also produce HORMONES which are passed into the BLOOD STREAM. Although these circulate all round the body they CONTROL functions "LOCAL" to the System which produced them :-
e.g. STOMACH { GASTRIN, GASTROZYMIN }

SMALL INTESTINE { ENTEROGASTRONE, SECRETIN, PANCREOZYMIN, CHOLECYSTOKININ, VILLIKININ }

Although each ENDOCRINE GLAND has specific functions all are interdependent. Overactivity or Underactivity of any one of them affects the whole system.

Figure 54

Attitude to **mental stress**, the pressure one chooses to have, determines whether uncontrolled adrenalin is released. In enjoyment or positive stress, such as dancing, adrenalin output is controlled and regulated. In anxiety or neurosism, liberation of adrenalin becomes uncontrolled and excessive. This could be detrimental to our well-being, involving embarrassment, "stage fright", palpitation, worry and tension.

Hardly any adrenalin is secreted under tranquil resting conditions. Therefore, assurance, encouragement or your own *determination to succeed* (with elation) is significant.

On the other hand, by increasing your opponent's adrenalin you have an added, if unfair, advantage, e.g., the behaviour of certain notable sportsmen.

A well-balanced diet

A well-balanced diet must contain the ingredients of protein, fat, carbohydrate, vitamins, minerals and water. Next to oxygen and water, protein is essential to life. During times of famine: absence of protein would first cause nutritional oedema (abnormal accumulation of fluid in the body with swollen abdomen) due to lowered blood-plasma protein, followed by death.

The role of protein

(1) Protein is a necessary constituent of all living human cells.
(2) It is absorbed as amino acids and is a source of energy for growth, repair and replacement of tissue cells, foremost amongst these are some 5,000,000 red blood cells and the average life of a red blood cell is about 3 weeks.
(3) It is essential for the formation of **enzymes** and **hormones**.
(4) If the constructive energy of protein matches that of tissue destruction, a state of metabolic equilibrium is reached. If in excess, i.e., more protein intake than is used up, then more nitrogenous waste products are excreted in the urine.
(5) Protein forms approximately 17% of body weight (fat about 12%; carbohydrate, less than 1%). More than 66⅔% of body weight is water.
(6) Minimum daily requirement of protein for an adult is about 40 gms.

The role of fat

(1) Fat is an inherent component of body cells, existing in high concentration in blood corpuscles' walls, ovaries and lactating breasts.

(2) It is necessary for bile production in the liver.

(3) Fat is needed for absorption of fat-soluble vitamins: A, D, E and K; otherwise these are lost in the excreta.

(4) It is 2¼ times more concentrated "energy fuel" than carbohydrate: 1 gm of fat liberates 9 calories compared with 4 calories for carbohydrate.

(5) It is readily stored as energy, forming about 12% of body weight: equivalent to 64,800 calories in a 60 kgms body (9½ stones or 133 lbs.).

(6) Fat is a carrier of food flavours and is a lubricant which helps swallowing.

(7) It is responsible for the comely smooth curvature of the female. It is the **excessive** intake of fat which is deleterious (as will be shown later).

The character of fat

Fat is present in the body in **two** entirely different forms: (a) **Depot** fat, mainly in the subcutaneous tissue, termed adipose tissue and around internal organs. It consists of connective tissue cells distended with neutral fat. The source of this fat is primarily the fat in the food. This is broken down by digestive **enzymes** into glycerine and fatty acids, carried into the blood stream to the cells to re-combine in different relation to form neutral human fat. The liver acts as an intermediary in the chemical process. If ingestion of carbohydrate is constantly excessive, the unused balance is converted into and stored as fat. Excessive fat deposit leads to **obesity**.

Proteins take no part in fat formation.

The curves of a woman's body and her rounded breasts are due to local accumulation of fat: adipose tissue. The active **ovaries** are essential for this curvature, though the pituitary indirectly influences the ovaries. The ovaries become fibrotic (scarred and contracted) after the menopause, usually near the age of 50 years. This natural pleasing appearance should not be confused with *excess fat*, particularly in the abdomen, both in the wall and in the **omentum**: a double fold of membrane passing from the stomach to other abdominal organs. **Slimming** achieves greater uniformity whilst the ovaries are still active.

(b) **Lipoids** (lipos = fat; eidos = resembling). They are fat-like substances, mainly **cholesterol** and its compounds. These are present in all cells, and in abundance in (i) the **bile** (chol = bile); (ii) the walls of the **blood corpuscles**; (iii) the **ovaries**, and at the end of a pregnancy there is an outpouring of cholesterol in the milk.

Increased intake of **cholesterol**, however, overburdens otherwise normal cells with excess lipoids, leading to fatty degeneration. The minute droplets of fatty degeneration fuse to form larger globules of fatty **infiltration**, which undermines the function of cells and their utilisation of oxygen. Toxins (poisonous substances) are also formed in the process.

The role of carbohydrate

(1) Carbohydrate is absorbed as glucose to circulate in the blood stream. The normal fasting blood glucose level is about 100 mgm per 100 c.c. of blood. Glucose is used in cell metabolism.

(2) It is the first and prime source of **muscular energy**, stored in the **liver** and skeletal **muscles** as glycogen. Larger muscles (trained) possess more glycogen than the untrained and have higher stamina. It is the progressively trained muscles which afford expansion of muscle fibres with protein and greater storage capacity of glycogen.

(3) Carbohydrate is necessary for the complete combustion of fat, otherwise toxic fat intermediaries such as aceto-acetic acid infiltrate the blood, liver and urine.

Dietary fibre

Dietary fibre is mainly a carbohydrate but **unaffected** by digestive enzymes. Enzymes are complex organic substances (compounds of carbon) secreted by various parts of the alimentary canal (the bowel) and act as catalysts: inducing chemical changes (digestion), themselves remaining unchanged. Fibre is present in different parts of plants such as husks, pods, seed coats and cell walls; detailed as follows:

(a) **Envelopes** of grains, not the grains themselves or their skin, but their stiff dry wrapping outer covering, removed before the grain is used as food. These are the husks or chaff, e.g., coarse **bran**.

(b) **Pods** of pulses, not the beans or peas themselves, e.g., the flat fleshy pods of runner beans enclosing the seeds.

(c) **Coats** of grains and pulses, the skin itself, termed pericarp.

(d) The microscopic **cell walls** of all edible plants. A cell wall, of cellulose (a carbohydrate), surrounds the nutrient protoplasm. The cell walls form the basis of all **vegetable** and **fruit** fibre. If these crops are unrefined they contain fibre in varying quantities: whole grain bread (8%), baked beans (7%), cabbage (2.5%), apple (2%), as against **bran** (44%).

A bulking agent

Dietary fibre functions as a bulking agent:

(i) Fibre-rich foods are retained longer in the stomach and digested more slowly. This discourages over-eating, over-nutrition and **obesity**.

(ii) A bulking agent stimulates peristalsis, the wave-like contraction of the intestinal wall, accelerating the **transit** of food residue. The effect is twofold: (a) lessens **constipation**; (b) decreases the formation of those "wayside pockets of ill-fame" called **diverticulosis**, and when inflamed, diverticulitis.

(iii) Colonic **bacteria** break down fibre. Bacteria of the colon rapidly multiply by the presence of fibre — they like it. Their action on fibre is not unlike that of fermentation effected by yeast on sugary solution. **Fermentation** is a chemical change induced by the action of a ferment, chemical or living, splitting the substance, eg., fibre, into simpler products. The fermentation here proceeds as follows: (a) **hydrogen** is liberated by the bacterial action on fibre $(CH_2O)_x$; (b) this hydrogen combines with **sulphur** (a residue of earlier protein digestion), to form **hydrogen sulphide** (H_2S) — an unpleasant smelling gas; (c) some methane gas (CH_4) is also formed in the fermentation process.

The bulky stools are made up of (a) enormous quantities of colonic **bacteria**; (b) fermented fibre which evolves **gas**; (c) unaffected fibre; (d) other food residue; (e) water. All result in soft bulky stools and gas. The motions should be soft but formed; if runny, intake of fibre should be reduced. The easy evacuation allays and lessens the incidence of **constipation**, **haemorrhoids** and **anal fissures**.

Vitamins and minerals

Vitamins (vita = life) are a group of substances present in natural foodstuffs, which are essential to normal metabolism, the lack of which causes deficiency diseases. A well-balanced diet with *cereals, milk,* **fresh** vegetables and fruit contains almost all the vitamins and minerals likely to sustain health. Except for the neglected very young and the aged, those with certain diseases, and those engaged in highly competitive sport, extra vitamins are superfluous. It is important to know merely which foods are rich in any particular vitamin(s) so that these are not excluded from the diet entirely. Vitamins are usually referred to alphabetically: **A, B$_{1-12}$, C, D, E, K.**

The role of minerals

The body has in its constitution the elements of iron, copper; calcium, phosphorus; iodine; potassium, sodium, chlorine. These are needed in minute but measurable quantities. Briefly their metabolism is as follows: **iron** is an essential constituent of haemoglobin of the red blood cells, **copper** aids their formation. **Calcium*** is the chief constituent of bone (calcium phosphate), necessary for adequate heart-muscle contraction, blood clotting, nerves' excitability regulation. **Phosphorus** is present in all cells and in high concentration in the *blood, brain* and *liver.* **Iodine** is necessary for the formation of thyroxin, the active principle of the thyroid gland. In districts where the iodine supply in the drinking water is insufficient, simple goitre can develop. **Potassium** is known to relax heart-muscle. **Sodium**

---

* Bone is hard tissue consisting mainly of **calcium** phosphate and carbonate, forming a dense compact outer layer (about ⅔rd of the bone, by weight), covered with a thin membrane (periosteum). The inner layer is spongy (about ⅓rd by weight), containing organic matter in its middle, termed bone **marrow**, which, in some long and flat bones, is largely concerned with **blood formation**. Amongst its functions, **calcium** is essential for ossification of bone and is absorbed from the bowel if in soluble form, as in milk, its products and green vegetables, along with **vitamin D**. Calcium is carried to the bones by the blood plasma, the liquid part of the blood. The average level of plasma calcium is 10mg per 100 c.c. (0.01%), dependent, amongst other factors, on the secretion of the parathyroid glands in the neck.

The diminishing of the ovarian hormone, **oestrogen**, at the menopause, could lead to loss of calcium from bones and consequent **osteoporosis** (porosity or rarefaction of bones making them less dense), leading to possible curving of the spine and fracture of bones. Soluble calcium, vitamin D and exercise that improves circulation and metabolism are significant to avoid brittle bones, in **men** as well as **women**. Alcohol, certain drugs, including cortisteroids (over a period) inhibit the utilisation of calcium in forming bone tissue.

maintains the rhythmic contraction of heart beat. Sodium chloride gives tissue fluid its proper osmotic pressure.

Other **trace** elements in the body include aluminium, chromium, cobalt, magnesium, manganese, molybdenum, selenium and zinc. Most trace elements enter into the formation of enzymes. Magnesium is necessary in the composition of chlorophyll which is present in all green vegetables. There is no evidence, however, that aluminium is beneficial. Tea is a known source of aluminium. Toxic trace elements in the body usually originate from pest-disease agrochemicals, food additives and drugs.

The initial source of all minerals is the soil, and they are absorbed by the plants. The body's natural mechanism maintains the normal levels, and any excess minerals' intake could disturb the digestive system.

The origin of minerals and vitamins

A plant's visible shoot above the soil, consisting mainly of the young stem and leaves, has a green pigment, **chlorophyll**, which is made up of protein. This chlorophyll may be truly said to be the "staff of life", since in its process of chemical synthesis is manufactured the **food** upon which the whole **animal kingdom** depends; carnivores are dependent on the protein (flesh) of herbivores.

This green pigment, in the presence of **sunlight***, takes up the carbon dioxide (CO_2) from the **air**, which, in combination with water (H_2O) present in the leaves through its absorption from the **soil** by the roots, forms glucose (C, H and O), a carbohydrate, whilst releasing oxygen into the air. The glucose subsequently changes into starch. The absorbed water contains the minerals a healthy plant needs. Man's supply of vitamins and minerals comes directly from plants or from animals fed on plants (cow's milk and meat).

The resemblance of carbohydrate and fat (for the technical)

Carbohydrate and fat possess resembling molecular formulas: glucose $C_6H_{12}O_6$; beef fat $C_{57}H_{110}O_6$; both have C, H and O atoms in their constitution, in the same proportion as water (H_2O) in the case of carbohydrate but not in fat. Protein, however, is a highly

---

* The manifestation of life is probably the product of the sun's radiant energy.

94

complex compound constructed from the amino-group, such as alanine (a decomposition product of protein), with the formula $CH_3.CH.NH_2COOH$. Many proteins also have sulphur in their composition.

Air and water are vital nutriments

Oxygen and water are vital for growth and metabolism. Life is impossible without them and over two-thirds of the body weight is water. Oxygen consumption is multiplied enormously on physical exertion.

Water enters into the composition of all bodily fluids including blood plasma, lymph, cerebro-spinal fluid and digestive juices. It provides all cells with fluid which contains the minerals, vitamins, hormones and enzymes. Metabolism would be impossible without oxygen and fluid.

Water balance

We tend to eat more and drink less (water) than we require. Healthy kidneys maintain the optimum fluid content of the blood and tissues and also the appropriate balance between water and minerals in accordance with the needs of the body. Even if 2 litres (3½ pints) of water were drunk in 15 minutes, urinary output would rise immensely and the 2 litres of water would be eliminated within the next 2 hours. At almost any time any excess fluid reaching the blood which cannot be excreted immediately (because of its quantity) by the kidneys, is temporarily accommodated in the *tissue spaces* of the liver, muscles, skin and kidneys. This temporary storage is effectively to maintain the normal **blood volume,** which is about 5 litres (8.8 pints) in a full-grown adult, and is about 1/11 of body weight. A bland non-alcoholic beverage such as tea, coffee, fruit drink, water, taken after muscular exercise is appropriate to compensate for water loss by the skin (perspiration), water-vapour expelled by the lungs and urinary secretion by the kidneys.

In considering a well-balanced diet, quality alone is not enough, quantity and frequency must be taken into account. The total intake of essential nutriments should balance with the amounts stored, used up as energy, lost as heat or excretion.

Chapter 12

QUANTITATIVE BALANCE OF NUTRITION

Measurement of metabolism

Nutrition is the taking and using of food for nourishment, and food is a source of **power**: which is energy that can be measured.

Calorie is the heat **unit** employed in the study of metabolism. It is the amount of heat required to raise a **kilogram** of water from zero to 1°C. This is sometimes called the larger calorie or kilocalorie.

The value of "calorie" as a unit of energy is to estimate how **much** and how **often** we need the various nutriments. Had the same weight of any food yielded the same worth of energy, there would be no need for the "calorie". Examples:

Type of food per 100 gm	Energy Calories	Percentage composition			Main Vita- mins
		Protein %	*Fat* %	*Carbo- hydrate* %	
Bread (wholemeal)	235 cal.	8	2.5	45	B
Cereal: Bran Flake	320	10	1	67	C, B
Milk	70	3.5	4	4.5	A, D, C
Butter	720	0.4	80	0.1	A
Cheese (Cheddar)	410	26	34	0.1	A, B
Eggs (boiled)	180	12	11	10	A, B
Sugar (white)	400	0.0	0.0	100	
Jam	200+	1	0.0	50	C trace
Marmalade	280	0.1	0.0	70	A, C
Chicken (roast)	150	25	5	0.1	B
Ham (boiled)	150	20	8	0.1	B
Lamb (roast)	180	28	7	0.1	B
Beef (roast)	200	29	9	0.1	B

Type of food per 100 gm	Energy Calories	Percentage composition			Main Vitamins
		Protein %	*Fat* %	*Carbo-hydrate* %	
Cod (grilled)	100	20	2	0.1	B
Potatoes (boiled)	90	1.5	0.1	20	C, B
Potatoes (baked)	110	2.5	0.1	25	C, B
Runner beans (boiled)	20	2	0.2	3	A, C, B
Baked beans	70	5	1	10	B
Cabbage (raw)	18	1.2	0.1	3	A, C
Tomatoes (fresh)	17	1	0.1	3	A, C
Lettuce	14	1.5	0.4	1.2	A, C, B
Apple	20	0.2	0.2	12	A, C, B
Orange (skinned)	40	0.8	0.1	9	C+,A,B

Physical exercise (energy release) per hour employs about 300 calories.

It is sensible to know the approximate caloric value of the nutriments we consume and release. By repetition, 50gm (2 large spoonfuls) of milk in a cup of coffee, repeated 5 times in a day means 35 calories multiplied 5 times or 175 calories daily. A 100 gm (3½ oz) serving of roast **beef** means 200 calories, whereas the same weight of roast **chicken** means 150 calories. If meat is repeated in one day, it could mean 350–400 calories for 200 gm. By daily repetition, you can guess the caloric value of food you eat without reference to tables.

Our daily calorie needs

Our calorie requirements change with **age**, surface area and physical **activity** (occupation and exercise). A **male** needs some 15% more than a **female**. A rough guide is as follows (daily):

Woman   2,000–2,400 calories
Man   2,300–2,775 calories

An athlete may need 3,000–4,000 calories

Metabolism can be **measured** scientifically for a given time by the amount of **oxygen** inhaled, **carbon dioxide** exhaled or **heat** produced or all three, since nutriments are combusted by O_2 in the tissues to produce $CO_2 + H_2O$ + heat + energy.

Individual caloric requirements can be calculated from height and weight by a given formula, but not taking into account the type of food, amount of exercise and last but not least the inherent quality and performance of the endocrine glands. The last-named often account for variation in loss of weight when all other factors appear identical between two individuals undergoing slimming. There are, of course, other biological variations, e.g., length and performance of the alimentary canal, which is about 8 metres (26 feet) in length during life, and time taken between ingestion and evacuation is about 20 hours.

Metabolism apportionment

Active metabolism	= **resting** metabolism	+ **added** metabolism
2,200 calories	= 1,500 calories	+ 700 calories

Active metabolism is taken to mean the chemical changes during activity: work energy, which is about 2,200 calories a day. It could be less for a sedentary occupation and more for moderate or heavy work.

Resting metabolism, also termed **basal** metabolism, is energy needed and used when a person is (a) at complete rest, physically and mentally but not asleep; (b) is not taking food, thereby no energy being used in digestion; (c) in a warm room. The energy calories required (input) and used (output) is approximately 1,500 calories daily.

Added metabolism suggests the difference between active and resting, which would be the product of skeletal muscular activity plus the extended chemical changes brought about by food stimulation, accelerated heart beat, circulation; respiration; digestion; peristalsis; secretion of kidneys; skin; endocrine glands; increased muscle tone during the day. This added metabolism is about 700 calories per day.

Nutriments-apportionment

Nutriments-apportionment of a well-balanced diet is determined by the requirements of: (1) Basal metabolism. (2) Stimulating effect of food and loss of energy in the excreta. (3) Muscular work. (4) Maintenance of the nitrogenous balance between (a) the production of new living cells (anabolism) and (b) the breakdown of cells (catabolism). Provision must also be made for the added new tissue formation in the **young**. In the elderly, a reduction of quantity, not quality, should be practised.

The ingredients-apportionment of a well-balanced diet is now suggested. It is for guidance only and capable of adjustment to suit a particular individual.

The daily average

Nutriment	Weight gm	Nutriment wt %	Cal per 1 gm	Total calories	
Protein	80	16.5	4.1	80×4.1	= 328
Fat	55	11.3	9	55×9	= 495
Carbohydrate	350	72.2	4	350×4	=1400
	485	100			2223

It will be observed that the 80 gms of protein represent only a percentage of an ingested food such as beef, and 29% only of beef's weight is absorbable protein (see list). A "275 gms" of beef yields 80 gms of protein ($275 \times \frac{29}{100} = 80$ gms). Similarly "68 gms" of butter yield 55 gms of absorbable fat ($68 \times \frac{80}{100} = 55$ gms). In a well-balanced diet there would be more than one protein-food. Nutriments percentages here (16.5% and 11.3%) are not unlike the weight percentages that exist in a healthy body. To sustain your health, movement and muscular exercise are necessary to utilise most of the carbohydrate.

Suggested slimming regimen

Assuming that there is no glandular abnormality or disease, a slimming diet could be as follows:

Commence with 1,500 calories a day for 3 days, gradually reduced to 1,000 (woman); 1,150 (man) by the end of the first week. Second week: 1,000 (1,150) daily. Third week: regulate between 1,000 and 1,500. Subsequent weeks: adjust intake. The **purpose** is to arrive at the correct weight for your sex, age and height and to establish the right weight. The object is to lose ½–1 kg (1.1–2.2 lb) per week. Your water intake daily (in coffee, milk, fruit drinks, plain water) should be 1½ litres (about 3 pints) but not less; any nutriments in drinks should be taken into the reckoning. The diet must be well-balanced to contain the necessary ingredients.

Over-eating is often habituated by the mind and the more you eat the more you want to devour. Commercial slimming diets basically depend for their temporary success on motivation, inducement or promptness to respond.

The initial loss will be tissue fluids before the depot fat is mobilised and released.

Keeping fit

In addition to a regular and regulated nutrition, keeping fit through muscular exercise (movement) will not only ensure the presence of protein and glycogen in your muscles for strength and stamina, but will determine the state of your (a) circulation; (b) oxygenation; (c) metabolism; (d) drainage of tissue waste-products. These are the pillars upon which the quality of life relies.

You can, of course, satisfy every craving for food, alcohol, tobacco, drugs and sensual desires, to avoid frustration. Such habits of the **mind** become addictive and devotional. Folly is stronger than reason. In this way, prepare for a future of grief. You are likely to have it.

Summary

This exposition began (Chapter 11) by unfolding the meaning of metabolism, which is the foundation of our understanding of a well-balanced diet to sustain health. It proceeded by explaining the factors which influence the chemical changes in the living body whether through nutrition, muscular exercise or hormones. It then adopted the following successive stages to enable the reader to judge what sort of diet is likely to secure health:
The meaning of a well-balanced diet
The roles of protein, fat and carbohydrate
The character of fat
Dietary fibre and its significance
Assessing vitamins and minerals and knowing their source
Water balance in the body
How metabolism is measured in calories and why
What are our caloric needs

Nutriments-apportionment in our diet
Assessing a slimming diet

THE AIM

It is not, of course, intended that you should memorise the foregoing details on the subject of "diet". You will not be likely to have the time or the inclination to do this, and, even if you did attempt it, the result would be to find yourself enmeshed in a huge web of particulars.

More to the purpose, these pages will acquaint you with the technical terms and the principles by means of which you will grasp the meaning of a well-balanced diet to secure health and joy. You will also be able to discern the rationality or otherwise of any dietary course you may be offered, in the knowledge that whatever it may be, you have the mental resources to judge it.

Effect of alcohol on metabolism

Over eighty per cent of the adult population of Great Britain drink alcohol. There is no question, however, that **alcohol** has the power to damage human fat including protoplasmic **lipoids**. Lipoids, chiefly of cholesterol, which are present in the cytoplasm, is the semi-fluid substance forming the basis of all body cells.

The injurious action of alcohol upon lipoids causes **fatty degeneration**: the cells first appear tarnished or speckled (phanerosis). If there is no allowance for recovery in terms of days or weeks between alcoholic indulgences, some cells proceed to degeneracy and **atrophy**. This means emaciation or wasting away, owing to poor oxygenation and the cells' inability to assimilate nutriments and their conversion into living substances (anabolism).

The atrophied cells are replaced by fibrous (scar) tissues. These intersect those which have escaped atrophy — a condition known as **cirrhosis** which has a nodular, hobnail-like appearance.

The organs most affected are, in this order: stomach, liver (a metabolic factory), brain with cerebral oedema, known as "wet brain", kidneys and heart. Amongst the morbid changes found at *autopsy** (the dissection and examination of a dead body to determine the cause of death) of **chronic alcoholics** are: *chronic gastritis*, featuring thickening of the stomach lining with its surface pitted with infected areas so as to present a nodular appearance. *Liver cirrhosis*, the liver is enlarged with cloudy swollen cells and intersected by scar tissue, marking the atrophied groups of cells. *Chronic interstitial nephritis*, which is accompanied by degenerative changes in the kidneys. *Arteriosclerosis*, where the arterial walls possess fatty streaks and heaped-up patches and ulcers in their lining. Calcium deposits occur in the thickness of the wall itself, making the arteries hard but **brittle**. *Heart* and *lungs* may appear mottled from fatty degeneration or cells" atrophy.

The taking of a "case history" by a medical examiner requires as much or more skill than the subsequent physical examination, and acc▓▓▓▓▓d patience are often well rewarded by the diagnostic value ▓▓▓▓ts obtained. The resultant effects of alcohol on the body o▓▓▓▓▓vé often masked the diagnosis of other diseases. Because of these, it is necessary to enquire into and obtain accurate information from the examinee on the *"Amount and kind of alcohol, tobacco and drugs (if any) per week"*.

Despite the ravages of alcohol, some regular drinkers elude premature death, but are rarely, if ever, free from some ailment or complaint or worsening of an accompanying disease. It is well to remember that almost all of us are provided with spare organs: two lungs, two kidneys, two cerebral hemispheres, even the liver has two large lobes (with two additional smaller ones).

This thought is offered as worthy of preservation. It is one of the sagest and saddest observations ever made: **"Hell is the truth seen too late"**.

Summary of the entire exposition follows.

---

* The author carried out several autopsies. He is also a former life assurance medical examiner for the "Prudential", "Legal and General", "Sun Life of Canada" and "Manufacturers Life".

Summary of the Entire Exposition

KEEPING FIT — A PLEASURE*

For what purpose does anyone want to keep fit? What bodily improvements, if any, are achieved?

One of the pleasures of life is physical exercise which keeps you fit. Good health is a condition of soundness or strength; a state of well-being and freedom from illness. Health is largely dependent fresh air (oxygen), warmth, diet and exercise, both **muscular** and **men** means adaptability to the environment in our struggle for

Purpose of keeping fit

(1) **Enjoyment**; the awareness and experience of fitness, embracing the joy of agility, balance, co-ordination, good posture, rhythm, flexibility, stamina and strength.

(2) **Self-confidence**. Skilful movement and regulated exercises, carried out in company with others, do much to preserve the appearance of **youth** and help to lose self-consciousness.

(3) **Community spirit**. Keeping fit in company provides an excellent opportunity for mutual understanding and co-operation.

(4) **Preserving good health**. Without a doubt the main purpose of "Keep Fit" is implicit in the title itself — the preservation of good health. The motor car and television deprive most of us of the physical activity needed for healthy existence. It is the **walking**, not the riding and the **movement**, not the watching, that the body needs most.

Bodily improvements by keeping fit

There is little doubt that a "Keep Fit" class or association is judged

---

* Extract from a paper specially prepared by the author for the Keep Fit Association — a national organisation.

by the quality of its exercises, whether in "movement" or "dance". Bodily improvements as a result of **regular** and **regulated** exercises are many and varied and include:

(1) A more **powerful heart** beat, most likely due to better coronary circulation (circulation in the heart muscles themselves).

(2) Improved **circulation**, not only of blood, but lymph, in the minute capillaries, with better lymph supply and drainage of tissues, accelerating **metabolism**. This is the process by which nourishing substances are built up into living matter or by which living matter is broken down into simple substances to produce energy.

(3) Increased **oxygen-carrying** power of blood, principally as a result of expanded oxygen intake of the lungs.

The above three are causative factors in the increased efficiency of all tissues including the whole musculature, whether **voluntary** (skeletal) or **involuntary** (smooth) musculature of the organs, notably the **diaphragm** (skeletal). This is continually active, and next to the heart, the most important muscle of the body.

It is well to realise that the bony framework, the skeleton, provides not only attachments for muscles, tendons and ligaments, but support for the body organs.

Efficiency is thus in the range of movement and leverage, co-ordination (in conjunction with the brain), flexibility of joints and tonicity of organs: all as a result of increased blood and lymph circulations and oxygenation.

(4) **Greater tolerance** to lactic acid which pours into the blood stream during vigorous muscular exertion. Although **protein** is the main chemical component of muscle tissue, it is the muscle **glycogen** (a carbohydrate) whose breakdown leads to the formation of lactic acid, undermining the **alkalinity** of the blood.* **Oxygen** has the ability to

---

* In the presence of oxygen, muscle glycogen is converted to $CO_2 + H_2O$ + heat + energy, during muscular movement. During vigorous exercise and oxygen insufficiency, glycogen is anaerobically converted to lactic acid, then to lactate by the alkaline blood, then to $CO_2 + H_2O$ + heat + energy only in the presence of oxygen. Which stage is reached and where, is dependent, amongst other factors, on the speed and extent of the exercise exceeding or otherwise, the oxygen provision.

overcome lactic acid. Increased oxygen leads to increased rate of removal of lactic acid from the blood, and the improved chemical interaction determines the speed of recovery from exertion of the trained muscles.

(5) Greater **effortless** strength as a result of increase in the performance and volume of muscles exercised. Bodily activities in daily life are performed by the **flexor** muscles of the front, rarely by the **extensors** of the back of trunk or limbs. Extension or stretching movements are observed in "Keep Fit" movements to produce better balance and posture.

(6) More economical and correctly directed movements in life accrue from muscular exercises in **co-ordination**.

No improvements or loss of **superfluous fat** can be accomplished overnight. **Continuity** as well as **proper training** and a strict but well-balanced **diet** are the hallmarks of achievement. All body functions are orderly and regulated. Disorderly nutrition is against the essence of nature. Correct and constant physical activity carries with it a feeling of well-being, both of which enhance the **quality of life**.

Caution

The **vital centres** of the brain which control all bodily functions, receive during unaccustomed muscular exercise, blood reduced in quantity (despite rise in blood pressure), depleted of oxygen and loaded with CO_2, which may lead to exhaustion, unconsciousness or expiration. Persons exhibiting a struggle for breath after a minor exercise should not attempt further muscular exercise at the time. Safety also lies in graduated exercises, involving slow progression of physical intensity. Effectiveness, born of knowledge and the experience of a trainer, will thus result.

Inactivity

To sum up, let us not underrate the seriousness of inactivity which spells bodily decline and mental decay, concurrent with ageing. Your physical and mental potentials are waiting to be released — why not express them? Such resources do exist and are capable of utilisation. "Restfulness is a quality for cattle; the virtues are all active, life is alert".

INDEX

FIT...

THROUGH
MOVEMENT AND DIET

DR. B. H. BARRADA

STRENGTH   STAMINA   SUPPLENESS
FOR   ALL

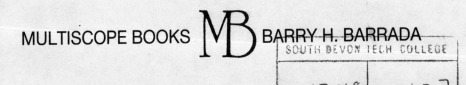

MULTISCOPE BOOKS **MB** BARRY H. BARRADA

By the same author

THE HUMAN COMPUTER in 3 concise volumes:
Volume 1: Instant Practical Steps. Expressions for Particular Usages. Memory. Voice. 192 pages.

Volume 2: Humour. Entertainment. Love. Repartee. Art of Persuasion. 240 pages.

Volume 3: Discourse—the Breath of Civilised Life (a verbal encyclopaedia). 288 pages.

Also: The Bare Essentials of the Human Computer—Extracts. 80 pages.

THE BARE ESSENTIALS OF HOW TO SUCCEED AS AN INVESTOR. 40 pages.

FITNESS FIRST THROUGH MOVEMENT AND DIET

ISBN   0–9510106–8–9

Copyright © H. Barrada 1988

ALL RIGHTS RESERVED

Printed in Great Britain by
A. Wheaton & Co. Ltd., Exeter, EX2 8RP
Typesetting by
Photoprint, Torquay, TQ1 1JD

Summary of the author's experience

Practised as

Artist
Cartoonist
Family doctor
Surgeon
Anaesthetist
Company managing director
Deviser of patent diagnostic instruments and appliances, and other registered designs
Local government councillor (independent)
Lecturer on First Aid, Taxation, Investment
Author
Freelance writer on diverse subjects
Organiser of Art Classes and Gardening Club

Author
Barry H. Barrada, M.B., Ch.B., M.R.C.S.(Eng.), L.R.C.P.(Lond.)

Also author of *MINITAX; INVESTMENT PROSPECTS* (Medstoc:Birmingham); *HOW TO SUCCEED AS AN INVESTOR* (Newnes:Lond.); *YOU AND YOUR MONEY*

MULTISCOPE BOOKS   MB   BARRY H. BARRADA

2 Mead Road, Torquay, Devon TQ2 6TE